Anticipating HEAVEN

Anticipating HEAVEN

SPIRITUAL COMFORT
and PRACTICAL WISDOM
for NAVIGATING LIFE'S
FINAL CHAPTERS

DR. PAMELA PRINCE PYLE

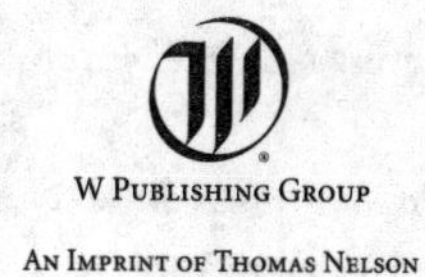

W PUBLISHING GROUP

AN IMPRINT OF THOMAS NELSON

Anticipating Heaven

Published in Nashville, Tennessee, by W Publishing, an imprint of Thomas Nelson.

Published in association with William K. Jensen Literary Agency.

ISBN 978-1-4003-4470-3 (audiobook)
ISBN 978-1-4003-4469-7 (eBook)
ISBN 978-1-4003-4445-1 (softcover)

Library of Congress Control Number: 2024940084

Printed in the United States of America

24 25 26 27 28 LBC 5 4 3 2 1

To my husband, Scott, whose love, support, and encouragement made this book possible.
To my family, who are loved more than they can imagine.
To my patients and friends, whose stories are told in these pages.
To my friend and agent, Bill Jensen, whose life story made this book what it is.

A NOTE OF THANKS

Each one of us has the capacity to impact others' futures for good. Nobel Peace Prize winner Mother Teresa of Calcutta exemplified that profoundly when she started The Missionaries of Charities in 1950. Its objective was to love and care for those who were marginalized in society and burdened with unmet needs. Her life impacted those she served and the millions who followed in her footsteps.

Another such person was Dr. Jim Towey, her trusted friend, advisor, and pro bono legal counsel. With Mother Teresa's encouragement, Dr. Towey formed the nonprofit advocacy organization Aging with Dignity in 1996 and Five Wishes, an advance care planning program, which has impacted over 40 million lives and provided foundational thoughts Anticipating Heaven.

I am exceedingly grateful to Dr. Towey, Paul O'Malley, and Joane Eason, the leadership of Aging with Dignity and the Five Wishes. They have been so generous with their time and the Five Wishes concepts appearing in this book. It is a joy to see the legacy of Mother Teresa continuing through their lives.

A portion of the proceeds of this book will be donated to Five Wishes in support of their work of health equity, end-of-life planning, and advocacy for aging with dignity. You can learn more about their work and resources at www.fivewishes.org and www.agingwithdignity.org.

To order Five Wishes at my website, visit www.drpamela.com. Perhaps your fifth wish will include a legacy inspired by Mother Teresa and build toward a future even she could not have envisioned.

—Dr. Pamela Pyle

CONTENTS

Foreword xi
Preface xiii

PART 1: PREPARING YOUR PLAN

Chapter 1: An Unexpected Question 3
Chapter 2: An Unanticipated Reality 9
Chapter 3: When in a Foreign Land 27
Chapter 4: Diminishing Chaos 47
Chapter 5: A Bargain and a Treasure 59
Chapter 6: The Hard Hard Choices 71
Chapter 7: Care and Caring 89

PART 2: PREPARING YOUR MIND, HEART, AND SOUL

Chapter 8: Paradigm Shifts: Anticipating Heaven in the Storm 103
Chapter 9: The Final Paradigm Shift: "Wow, This Is It!" 125
Chapter 10: The Power of Prayer in God's Sovereign Care 145
Chapter 11: Hope amid Suffering 157
Chapter 12: The Most Important Preparation 171
Chapter 13: A Good Death 181

Acknowledgments 191
Further Practical Resources 195
Resource A: When Decisions Should Be Shared 196
Resource B: Guide to Documents and Advance Planning 200
Resource C: Understanding Brain Death 203
Resource D: Understanding Persistent Vegetative State 205
Resource E: Planning for Peace Checklist 206
Resource F: End-of-Life Timeline Signs and Symptoms 219
Resource G: The Dictionary of Serious Illness Terms 221
Notes 231
About the Author 237

FOREWORD

I have devoted my life to becoming a leader who adds value to other leaders, that they may add value to those they lead. Early in this journey I discovered that to succeed in this God-given purpose, I must remain a student of life and of those whom I teach.

As my journey has intersected with the lives of others, I have met many who have been called for a God-given, specific purpose and utilize the gift of lifelong learning to equip themselves and those they are called to serve.

Dr. Pamela Prince Pyle is one of these, and she's the author of the book you are about to read. As a physician for more than three decades in hospital-based medicine and as a medical missionary in Rwanda, Dr. Pamela has always considered her patients and their families invaluable lesson givers.

Her strong Christian faith and God-given empathy have inspired her to share the valuable lessons we all need when we face a serious or terminal diagnosis. She even teaches us how to prepare in advance of that diagnosis so there may be less chaos and fear in our final season.

As I read the story that inspired this book, I was captivated by the human drama unfolding as if I were in the room with her and her patient. Lessons emerge from her powerful mastery of storytelling and the lives of those who inspired those stories. From the practical lists of questions to ask your clinician to the undeniable power of faith amid a medical crisis, these lessons are those we don't even realize we need . . . until we do.

I encourage you to read this book with the mindset of a student and the heart of a teacher. What you are taught in *Anticipating Heaven* will benefit you now and later. You may become the messenger of lifelong learning and share the hope of living and dying while anticipating heaven.

In the words of one of her patients, "No one makes it out of here alive." With a chuckle, this patient teaches the essence of *Anticipating Heaven.* In the words of Dr. Pamela, "Keep your eyes eternally fixed as your feet are firmly rooted in the present."

I foresee this book becoming an evergreen resource for you and those you love. Bring Kleenex and a journal to take notes while you read this treasure of a book from my good friend, Dr. Pamela.

May God bless you and yours,
Dr. John C. Maxwell

PREFACE

Dear Reader,

You have been in my thoughts, prayers, and heart from the moment I began writing this book. I imagine you as those with whom I have sat face-to-face as we discussed a new diagnosis, a serious illness event, a terminal disease, the dying process, an impending death, or the tragedy of the unexpected.

You will read some of these patients' stories in these pages, most of whose names have been changed. The conversations recounted in the patient stories are not exact quotes but reflect the spirit of the words spoken.

I consider it a privilege for my life to intersect with the lives of those whose suffering leads to crucial conversations. Entering the suffering of another human being has taught me the courage of the human will, the resilience of the human spirit, and the capacity for love of the human heart. My patients and their families have been the wisest of teachers.

Wisdom's true value is found when it transcends one human life and positively impacts another. In over three decades of medical practice, I have shared this wealth of wisdom received from each life that crossed with mine and gifted it to the next convergence of lives I experienced. While you may be reading this in some distant place or time, I write to you as if we are within arm's reach. At this moment, our lives touch. Thank you.

Uniting faith and medicine changes how we approach life and death. The prospect of facing our own mortality teaches us about the brevity of life. This would summarize the wisdom of the patient stories in this book and the thousands of others I have witnessed.

But in this fleeting life, what happens if a health crisis arrives? What happens if life now has a time stamp? What do you do when the terminal illness isn't the sad story you talk about over family dinner, but it is your story, and no one feels like eating dinner?

It happens every second of every day!

If you are reading these words and *the second* is your second, you are in the right place. If you are reading these words and the empty chairs at the family dinner table are yours and your loved ones', you are in the right place. This book is written to patients and their loved ones.

But those who care for patients and families in a healthcare storm will also benefit. Healthcare workers, end-of-life providers, chaplains, caregivers, pastors, and church members will find this book to be a faith-filled resource for their service and work. Thank you for what you do.

How to Use This Book

I want to equip you with wisdom to help you become an advocate for your health or the health of someone you love. The principles you will learn in *Anticipating Heaven* are timeless and can be applied to different healthcare delivery systems.

The first half of the book is titled "Preparing Your Plan." It is greeting you wherever you are in the healthcare journey, whether you're a patient or your loved one is. It is the knowledge you need if you have just received a serious diagnosis or are living with one at the end. It equips you with the right questions at the right time, what to expect at the hospital, and knowledge to replace fear. It also helps you *live with the end in mind* and teaches you the importance of a plan to minimize chaos in times of catastrophe.

I share why it is important to begin with an advance care plan even when healthy and then walk you through how to complete one. The stories will prepare you for the nuances that come with making decisions and for the hard times that may come.

The second half of the book is titled "Preparing Your Mind, Heart, and Soul." As I walk you through the patient journey, we will talk about preparing your mind: how to find a good doctor, live with a chronic illness or disability, and be comforted until your last breath.

Your heart will be prepared and receive hope through the power of prayer in patient stories and the one prayer that *always* results in a miracle. You will be inspired by the faithfulness of God, even in suffering. He will intimately meet you in your time of need.

Your soul will be comforted by spiritual truths. You will read about the most important preparation before your last breath. Finally, you will read the story of a woman who taught me to anticipate heaven in the middle of the storm and who truly died a good death.

The "Further Practical Resources" section included at the end of this book contains helpful glossaries, checklists, and bonus information to work through and apply to your own situation. These resources have been curated to bring you the precise and concise information needed to understand medical jargon, medical decision-making, and medical planning. You will find them useful if you are navigating healthcare for your loved ones or yourself and looking to implement the guidance in this book right away. For instance, I highly recommend beginning your Planning for Peace Checklist, regardless of your health status. Taking care of the business end of dying gives more time to live while dying. This creates space for more love and fewer regrets.

This book is meant to be read in its entirety the first time. It will give you answers to the questions you already have. It will also give you questions to seek answers for what you need to know. Bookmark sections you may not need now but could at a future time. It will become a practical resource when you need it most.

In this book you will receive many tools to help you cope, but the greatest gift I wanted to bring you is hope. Hope comes through the practice of *Anticipating Heaven*.

We are each on a collision course with death. We don't know when that impact will occur. Our final chapters may be in the future, or we may be living in them now. Anticipating heaven brings clarity to life and the seconds that are here now and then vanish.

I pray that you are blessed by the spiritual comfort and practical wisdom you will receive in this book. Thank you for being here. You matter to me, and you matter to God.

In Christ,
Dr. Pamela

Part One

PREPARING YOUR PLAN

one

AN UNEXPECTED QUESTION

Every man must do two things alone; he must do his own believing and his own dying.
MARTIN LUTHER

I paused outside her closed door to catch my breath and gather my thoughts. Entering her room, I expected to find multiple family members surrounding her, as there had been on most days. Instead, she was alone.

As I shut the door behind me, the noises of a full ward faded, giving way to the gentle sounds of a humidifier and an elderly woman's labored breaths. Her eyes were closed, and an oxygen mask covered her nose and mouth. I glanced at the windowsill, where multiple cards were displayed—a child's drawing peeking out of one. Flowers were on the bedside table, with a family photo nearby. This was a well-loved woman.

I had witnessed her decline with each hospital visit, and it was obvious the end was approaching. She knew it, too, and had requested to speak with me that day. When I sat gently on the bed, her eyes opened. Recognizing me, her eyes revealed a faint smile underneath her mask. I reached for her hand and leaned forward so we might hear each other.

Her hand was frail in mine, yet her grip was tight as I began to share with her the painful truth: she was dying. Her disease had ravaged her lungs to the point that it was time to make some critical decisions.

She asked a series of straightforward and thoughtful questions, each one requiring her to gasp for air.

"So, how much time *do* I have left?"

"When I am short of breath like this, I feel terrible. Will my suffering worsen?"

"You've witnessed the final moments of many others. What will they be like?"

"My family understands what is coming, but what exactly will they see?"

In my thirty-three years of medical practice—in state-of-the-art hospitals in the United States and in more nascent clinics in Rwanda—I have had countless end-of-life conversations. Yet this was the first time a patient, friend, or family member asked such direct questions.

I answered her questions as clearly, honestly, and gently as possible. But something about this moment—perhaps her quiet strength in the face of imminent death, or maybe the fact that she would be missed terribly by her family, as well as by me—moved me unexpectedly.

When I finally said, "I'm so sorry to have to tell you these things," I began to weep.

To my surprise, my patient grabbed my other hand and squeezed even tighter. "It's okay," she said as she comforted me. "I am going to have *a good death*. Please prepare my family. I am ready."

As I left her room, the statement "I am going to have a good death" lodged in my mind. In the days and weeks that followed, I could not shake it. Sinking into my subconscious, the phrase sometimes woke me in the night, prompting me to wonder, *What does it mean to have a good death?*

I thought about how so many people struggle mightily against our common destiny, seeing nothing about it as good. Meanwhile, others face death willingly, almost eagerly, as though they are arriving at a long-sought destination or getting a chance at last to become the self they knew they were meant to be.

Here is something I know as a doctor: persistent pain is always a signal that deeper investigation is warranted. Maybe a question that will not go away is meant to serve the same purpose.

The Glorious Secret

Though we are always *sad*, we are never really *shocked* when death takes an elderly loved one or when we attend the funeral of a friend or neighbor who had suffered from chronic illness or long-term disability.

But then there are those other deaths. The out-of-order deaths that rip at our hearts. They cause us to look to our Creator and cry out, "Why?" We sob when a child dies. "This isn't how life is supposed to work!"

Persistent pain is always a signal that deeper investigation is warranted. Maybe a question that will not go away is meant to serve the same purpose.

Likewise, we struggle to accept the sudden passing of a young parent who has small children. And how are we to make sense of death when it comes via a senseless act of violence, up to and including the horrors of genocide? Perhaps you think—with good reason—that trying to find *good* in the wake of such *bad* is a fool's errand.

A good death? What possible good can be found in death? And yet my breathless patient who inspired my search for an answer was genuinely peaceful as she prepared to depart this life. She seemed to possess a great secret that might benefit those she was leaving behind.

Because of God's mercy in my own life, I *knew* her secret—and it was glorious. But it was not until I began to write about it that I truly learned to *live* her secret. This was a woman who was confident of her destination. This was a woman who lived a life *anticipating heaven.*

Most people have heard the old quip "The only certainties in life are death and taxes." But until that heart-stopping moment when Death raps loudly on the door, barges into one's hospital room, or whispers softly from the other end of a dreaded phone call, taxes seem like the surer reality. We indulge in fallacies: "If I don't think about death, maybe it'll forget about me." Or we entertain fantasies like, "I don't have to worry about that now. I've got at least thirty, maybe even forty years left."

Then reality hits. The fact that you are reading this book may mean that Death has pulled up a chair at your dinner table or has parked in a loved one's driveway. Maybe the grim specter of "the end" is the ignored elephant in the room. For those facing the ultimate loss (either their own life or the life of a loved one), this giant, uninvited, and unwelcome visitor has a way of hovering in the imagination, haunting one's every step and invading one's nightly dreams.

Realizing that we cannot escape it forever, we wonder, *Is there any way to lessen death's sting?*

From my experience as a doctor, I want to help you prepare for the unexpected difficulties that come with having a serious diagnosis and those that lead to end-of-life realities. You will receive the practical advice you need to navigate the foreign challenges of the healthcare system. This may impact how you care for your loved ones or how you make choices for yourself.

But the greater gift I hope you will receive in this book is from the Lord himself, through his inspired Word. He alone can bring you comfort through his Holy Spirit, enabling you to reject death's sting and instead discover what it means to live *anticipating heaven*.

> *Peace I leave with you, My peace I give to you; not as the world gives do I give to you. Let not your heart be troubled, neither let it be afraid.*
>
> JOHN 14:27

two

AN UNANTICIPATED REALITY

Hope is the thing with feathers—
That perches in the soul—
And sings the tune without the words—
And never stops—at all.
EMILY DICKINSON

She was gorgeous, with long, blonde hair that was the envy of all her friends. While typically such beauty is intimidating to other women, Julie's external beauty was overshadowed by her inner attractiveness. She was a warm, generous soul. As a result, she enjoyed a rich life centered on her faith, family, and countless friends.

Julie became a mother in her thirties and managed to balance a career and family life with unusual grace. In fact, she eventually found pleasure in mentoring young mothers as *they* struggled to juggle the responsibilities of work and home. By age forty, she had two beautiful school-aged daughters, and she stayed busy volunteering and managing all the roles of her life.

When Julie began to feel excessively tired, she did not think it unusual. She attributed her weariness and occasional dizziness to her hectic schedule (and perhaps her age). But one night, while getting up from the dinner table, Julie blacked out and fell. Her head narrowly missed the countertop. Her husband, Jeff, jumped up to catch her without success.

"Julie! Julie!" he shouted. The girls began to cry. Julie said later she could hear their voices as if at the end of a tunnel. She struggled for what seemed like minutes (though it was only seconds) to lift her heavy eyelids. When they slowly fluttered open, her husband's worried face was hovering over her. Her teary-eyed, scared girls stood visibly shaken just behind him.

"I'm okay," she mumbled. "I think I just stood up too fast. I must be tired or dehydrated, or both." Seeing the fear in her family's faces, she tried to sit up and comfort them with hugs. Jeff told her to lie down and started to call 911. Julie talked him out of it.

"No, don't call an ambulance. I'm feeling better. Really. I just have been going too hard, and I stood up too quickly. I'll take it easy tonight and call the doctor tomorrow. If she wants me to come in, I will, I promise."

Jeff agreed to this compromise, and the four of them then cuddled on the couch, watching a movie together. Julie would later remember that night as "the night of innocence." A night spent blissfully unaware of the path they were about to walk.

The Unwelcome Visitor

Julie's go-to physician was her obstetrician/gynecologist, the doctor who had delivered both her daughters. She was able to get in the very next day. As she described her symptoms, she mentioned some abdominal discomfort she had been having off and on for perhaps three months. She had found minimal relief taking antacids. "It's not a pain," she explained. "More of a bloated feeling, a dull ache. It's hard to describe."

The doctor asked a few more questions, and Julie admitted to not having much of an appetite. The doctor recommended blood work, and they scheduled a follow-up in two weeks.

Imagine Julie's surprise when she got a call two days later saying the doctor wanted to see her as soon as possible. Her lab results were concerning, the doctor said. Julie was profoundly anemic and had blood in her stool. She needed more blood work and a gastroenterology consultation.

The next three weeks were a blur (even more than usual) as Julie and Jeff shared the care of their daughters and went from one medical appointment to the next. Through all the additional tests and consultations, uneasiness grew into full-blown anxiety. Most nights they found Fear piled up on the couch with them, an unwelcome visitor.

On a sweltering Southern day—the sort of day on which Julie normally would have taken her girls to the beach—the couple found themselves sitting nervously in the office of a specialist. They were waiting for the results from a test earlier that morning. The doctor had asked that they both be there to discuss the results. Julie noticed as the doctor entered the room that he seemed to be shuffling his papers quite a bit, looking down, and avoiding eye contact. Finally, he cleared his throat nervously and said softly, "I'm sorry to have to tell you this, but your biopsy results are consistent with cancer."

What Julie heard was, *Cancer! Cancer! Cancer!* Stunned, she looked at her husband, as if to say, *Why is he screaming at us?* She then realized that the screaming was her own thoughts skittering around her mind. She had been hoping that the C word would never become *her* word—her wife, mother, young-busy-life word. Shocked, she sat back in a daze, noticing for the first time the black second hand ticking its way around the clock just above the doctor's head. She could see the doctor's lips moving, but all her faculties of hearing and processing and questioning were temporarily disabled.

Cancer.

That night, Julie and Jeff held hands in the dark, crying and praying, and crying and praying some more, until they were all out of tears and all out of words. Her final thought before sleep? *If only I had known . . .*

Anticipating Death

Cancer, amyotrophic lateral sclerosis (ALS), heart disease, pulmonary fibrosis . . . incurable, hospice, comfort care . . . death. Death! As a human being, your mind is drenched in these words and their implications.

You resist the words, yet your mind lingers upon them, twisting and turning them, attempting to give them a less devastating meaning. Reality ultimately straightens them, and you drag your thoughts across their bristled edges.

You go about your day, and your words and motions exhibit the strength of character and will for which you have been known. Perhaps, however, the ones closest to you notice in your smile a quiver of your lips or a glisten in your eyes. The body can't help but betray the fear that overwhelms you at times. After all, it has betrayed you with this disease and its bristly words.

You begin to *anticipate death.*

As a hospitalist—a doctor who practices in a hospital—I frequently saw people amid crises related to advanced illnesses. These patients are often experiencing a rapid decline in health. They (and their families) are almost always terrified by what is unfolding, and they feel helpless in their shock.

Sometimes people with chronic illness reach a point when the disease starts to trigger one complication after another. This is when fear often creeps into the patients' eyes. They know things are not going well, yet they may refuse to acknowledge to others, or even to themselves, what lies ahead.

Many patients who are nearing the end are unprepared to hear such news, even when the evidence and their bodies are loudly telling them the painful truth.

In my own medical practice, I found that patients and their families have more peace when they understand the diseases they are facing. Experts in medical ethics confirm my anecdotal observations. One study reported that 99 percent of patients want to know about their condition and believe their doctor is obligated to inform them. Some 95 percent agree that the course of a disease "is easier and the outcome is better" when they are informed and are allowed to play an active role in their treatment decisions.[1] The key words in those statistics are *informed* and *active.* Despite fear, it's better to be informed.

An Unknown Course

We were on a three-hour road trip. My husband, Scott, was "driving" a self-driving car, our friend Jerry sat in the passenger seat, and

I was in the back. Jerry was trying to reel in his fear from taking his first-ever ride in a self-driving car. Some people get quiet when they are filled with conflicting emotions. Jerry gets funnier. His one-liners had us laughing deep belly laughs.

But after a while the mood in the car became more serious. Jerry, a brilliant scholar and author, shared an event that occurred in his family a few years prior. Doctors had diagnosed his son Nicholas with cancer. Like it was to Julie and Jeff, the shock of their son's diagnosis of cancer was overwhelming to Jerry and his wife, Cindy.

Even though we may know intellectually that such crises happen to families every day, nothing prepares us for the moment when an emergency hits home. When it does, the moment is stamped indelibly on our hearts. We remember where we were, what we were wearing, what scent was in the air, and the exact time on the clock hanging just above the doctor's head.

In a flash that imaginary yet reliable anchor tying us to the life we have always known is gone. Suddenly untethered, we are lashed about, heading out on an unknown course. Or perhaps this feels more like crashing into a brick wall. Either way, life as we know it has changed forever.

While waiting to see the first cancer expert, Jerry and Cindy did what most people in the information age do: they scoured the internet for help, answers, and statistics on survival success. They sought hope through numbers, but the numbers they found were dismal.

Their first oncology visit confirmed their fears. They were told their son's cancer had a 35 percent survival rate.

They chose to seek another opinion, which is always advisable with any new and serious diagnosis. A second older and more experienced oncologist stated that, in his experience, normal treatment had shown a 65 percent chance of long-term survival! Because Jerry and Cindy took the time to ask their long list of questions, they left a little more encouraged. Staying informed translated to peace and hope. But how do you know what questions to ask?

The Right Questions at the Right Time

Everyone has different concerns when grappling with a frightening new diagnosis. If you or your loved one has received a serious diagnosis, it is important to have the questions ready. Julie and Jeff were caught so unaware when they first met with the doctor that questions eluded them.

The questions below are a framework for *the right questions at the right time* for a cancer patient. Aspects of these questions could be applicable for any serious diagnosis. Depending on the patient and the situation, you will likely want to know the answers to most or all the following questions.

THE BIOPSY REVEALED CANCER.

- Could you give me my diagnosis in writing?
- I want to fully understand my diagnosis and prognosis. Could you advise me on what to expect?
- Will I need to have other tests to confirm the diagnosis or to determine the stage of my cancer/disease?
- What tests will need to be done to evaluate this?
- How long will I have to wait for these tests and results?
- Is this a type of cancer/disease you treat frequently?

If not, are there cancer/disease treatment centers that specialize in my type of illness?

- Why do you think I have this type of cancer/disease? Is there a genetic predisposition to my disease? Should my family be tested?
- I would like to keep a physical copy of all my records, including biopsy results and any imaging scans that I have. What is the best way to obtain these?
- When will we have our next appointment?
- Is there anything else I should have asked and didn't?

THE RESULTS ARE IN.

- What are the different stages of this cancer/disease, and what do they mean?
- What is my grade and stage of cancer/disease?
- What is my prognosis based upon the stage and the type of cancer/disease that I have?
- What are my treatment options?
- What are the potential side effects from each of these treatment options?
- Where would I receive treatment?
- How soon do I need to begin treatment?
- Will other doctors be involved in my care?
- Is molecular testing available for my cancer/disease?
- Are there blood tests that you follow over time for my cancer/disease?
- Is there a possibility of curing my cancer/disease?

- What does remission or a cure look like from your perspective?
- How will treatment affect my daily life?
- Will this diagnosis affect my ability to have children?
- What can I do to help myself during treatment? Which resources do you recommend for diet, exercise, and so on?
- Are there complementary or integrative medicine therapies I should consider?
- Whom do I speak with about the financial aspect of treatment?
- How do I reach you or your clinical staff if I have additional questions between appointments?
- Is there anything I should be attentive to during treatment that I should report to you or your staff?
- If I were your family member, what would you recommend?
- I would like to seek a second opinion. I will need all my records so they can make as thorough an assessment as you have. Please do not take this personally, but as my own health advocate I want to be thorough.
- Is there anything else I should have asked and didn't?

TREATMENT HAS STARTED.

- I am having these symptoms. Are they related to the cancer/disease or the treatment?
- What can be done to help alleviate these symptoms?

- How do you feel the cancer/disease is responding to treatment?
    - If responding well: How would you assess my prognosis considering this?
    - If not responding well: Will you change my treatment regimen? What alternatives do I have? Why do you believe the treatment isn't working? Would I be a candidate for a clinical trial? Are there any treatment centers I should consider that focus on cancers/illnesses like mine?
- Do you see anything of concern in my bloodwork or images that may be adverse effects of my treatment?
- I am dealing with fear/anxiety/depression because of my cancer/disease. Are there support groups or a mental health counselor that you recommend?
- Is there anything else I should have asked and didn't?

SUCCESSFUL TREATMENT IS COMPLETED.

- What is my prognosis now?
- Am I cured or in remission?
- Will I continue to take medicine, and if so, for how long?
- How many years without my cancer/disease will it be before you consider me to be cured?
- How can I best care for myself between appointments? What warning signs should I be attentive to that would require scheduling an earlier appointment?
- What does follow-up look like?

- Is there anything I can do to keep my cancer/disease from returning?
- Are there any long-term consequences of my treatment for which I need to be observed?
- Is there anything else I should have asked and didn't?

TREATMENT IS NOT SUCCESSFUL.

- What next?
- Why do you think the treatment was not successful?
- Should I seek another opinion?
- Are there clinical trials that I would be a candidate for in this circumstance?
- What is my prognosis now?
- Is there still a possibility of cure?
- I want to be fully informed. I need to know if you believe that my condition is terminal and that I should consider hospice.
- If I were your family member, what would you recommend? If you were me, what would you do?
- Is there anything else I should have asked and didn't?[2]

Jerry and Cindy asked their questions of the second doctor, then they chose to consult a *third* experienced clinician, which resulted in yet another prognosis. Looking at the same child, the same cancer, the same lab results, and the same treatment options, this doctor felt strongly that Nicholas had a 100 percent chance of long-term survival, and he promised that if anything ever changed in his prognosis, he would promptly inform them.

I am sure you would choose as Jerry and Cindy did. Nicholas began care with the third doctor. Jerry, Cindy, and Nicholas remained informed and active in the decisions regarding treatment. Today, many years later, Nicholas experiences good health.

Not every story ends like this. But this family's decision to seek more than one opinion in the face of a serious illness was wise. And do not minimize the hope offered by doctor number three. When the family was trying to stay afloat amid waves of despair and hopelessness, the third doctor threw them a lifeline.

Your doctor will be your main source of information. Yet if you or your loved one has been diagnosed with a serious illness, you may wonder what else you can do to stay informed and what the best way is to be informed. How do you actively make choices between therapies and treatments?

Living in the information age is both a blessing and a curse. Dr. Google will report millions and sometimes billions of results (the search term *cancer* has 4.79 billion at the time of this writing). There is a staggering amount of scientific knowledge only a few clicks away.

But it is difficult for the average person to know when to self-diagnose and treat and when to seek care from a clinician. It gets more challenging if you get your information about your disease process only from the internet.

I have discovered that this wealth of information is a helpful resource *after a person has a definitive clinical diagnosis.* But it is important to complete a vetting process for each website you look to for information.

- Nonprofit organizations such as www.cancer.org are generally credible. Look for: websites that end with *.org*, *.gov*, or

.edu. These represent nonprofits, government entities, and education centers, respectively.

- Avoid websites with a commercial bias. A website may have content about cancer and yet focus on one therapy, which they are selling.
- Evaluate the motivation or purpose of the website. Is it marketing or educational? The "About Us" or "About This Site" section frequently speaks to the motivation.
- Consider the science. It is easy to promote "scientific research" when, in fact, there is very little resembling science. A valid study will be easily accessible and transparent about its sourcing. It will discuss key components of the scientific method used: making an observation, forming a hypothesis, making a prediction, and analyzing results. Peer-reviewed articles add validity.

  Another method to evaluate a study is placement in a medical or scientific journal. Look at footnotes to determine the source of information. If sources have been published in journals that include articles on other topics, it is more likely a valid study. Ask your clinician if you still have doubts.
- Proceed with caution when you see claims of a secret ingredient, scientific breakthrough, miracle cure, or ancient remedy. Also beware when a money-back guarantee is offered or when one product treats multiple issues.

Even if you proceed cautiously, knowledge, in the absence of wisdom, can be difficult to interpret at best and harmful at worst. Try combining the wisdom of a trusted clinician with the information from reliable online resources—that will help you and your loved ones to become your best health advocates.

The Good Word

Once Julie was diagnosed with cancer, Julie and Jeff clung to each other in the first doctor's appointment and all the days that followed. At that moment, they could not fathom a life with a time stamp. No one had seen this coming. Normalcy had been disrupted, and they were facing a sudden detour onto an unfamiliar, twisty path with an unknown destination. Trepidation and fear are inevitable in situations like these.

Julie and Jeff chose to seek a second opinion at a respected cancer center. They were more prepared for the second doctor visit. The couple sat across from a doctor who confirmed Julie's diagnosis, but then he offered more hope in terms of specific treatment options. Julie quickly came to trust and like this new doctor.

Though still fearful, she and Jeff found comfort in leaving with a plan. While her diagnosis certainly interrupted their lives, having a plan allowed Julie to continue to be who she was: wife, mother, and friend. More importantly, she found a new and better word to replace the C word that had previously terrified her—the word *hope*.

Looking for Hope

Hopelessness kills, if not physically, then emotionally and spiritually. I consider it vital for clinicians, family members, and friends to speak hope to those who are struggling with debilitating and terminal illnesses. Patients need to know where to look for hope.

Hope comes in many forms to patients and loved ones: hope they will receive the best care possible, hope for a cure (or at least a few extra months or years), hope for a decent quality of life, hope for less pain, hope that loved ones and friends will stay close till the end, hope that one's suffering might be minimal, hope that one's life and legacy will make a lasting difference. In this regard, hope extends to those left behind: hope for their futures, hope for comfort from their grief, hope that their lives will turn out not just okay but happy.

I have noticed that some end-of-life patients who have been previously convinced this life is all there is begin to rethink their views. Some begin to hope they have been wrong. Others steel themselves in hope of the nothingness they believed in—"Ashes to ashes, dust to dust."

Ultimately, as patients understand that their days are numbered, those who find the greatest peace are those who have genuine hope in what comes next. They confidently expect a life beyond death, a life free of suffering, a world where, to paraphrase author J. R. R. Tolkien, everything sad is going to come untrue.[3]

Hope has a bigger purpose, a greater calling. Hope is a source of strength that enables you to continue by focusing the mind on a future minute, hour, day, life, or eternity that is different from your current momentary circumstance.

Hope. Hope. Hope. What a beautiful word for anticipation.

Those who find the greatest peace are those who have genuine hope in what comes next.

Julie added many new words and phrases to her medical glossary during the next two years. They were terms like *chemotherapy, immune suppression, radiation therapy, palliative therapy, alternative therapy, nutritional therapy, metastasis, failure of therapy, comfort therapy,* and *hospice.*

Stop. Stop. Stop.

One day near the end, she stared out the window, awed by the clouds in the sky and listening to the beautiful notes of "Clair de Lune." In that moment her final word became evident. *Hope.*

Going Home

Julie's journey, which began with her saying, "If only I had known," drew to a close with her knowing the most important things. She knew the love of her Savior and the reunion to come. She experienced the wonder of a loving family and friends, the marvel of music, the magnificence of a cloudy sky that had never been before and would never be again. She believed in the power of faith and hoped it would blossom in her daughters. Despite her sadness, she saw it all clearly. Life with hope is beautiful, and beauty is good.

I was on my way home from taking my son to camp when Jeff called. Julie had passed away that morning. I imagined the scene. Julie was surrounded by family in her home, *going home.*

Julie taught me a lot during her short life. She was a true friend. I loved her deeply and miss her fiercely. I find comfort in knowing her path.

This is the path we can travel. It is the path of life and dying and death while walking with *hope.*

Jeff and Julie experienced the "living hope" of Christ, and that changes everything.

> Blessed be the God and Father of our Lord Jesus Christ, who according to His abundant mercy has begotten us again to a living hope through the resurrection of Jesus Christ from the dead, to an inheritance incorruptible and undefiled and that does not

> fade away, reserved in heaven for you, who are kept by the power of God through faith for salvation ready to be revealed in the last time. (1 Peter 1:3–5)

In the pages to come, beyond the wisdom you need to navigate the healthcare system with your new words, you will find stories of hope. The Bible is God's Word. It is the ultimate story of hope. I pray amid the words you hear or read that you remember these words from our

Holy God.

> *When this corruptible has put on incorruption, and this mortal has put on immortality, then shall be brought to pass the saying that is written: "Death is swallowed up in victory."*
>
> 1 CORINTHIANS 15:54

three

WHEN IN A FOREIGN LAND

Knowledge is power.
SIR FRANCIS BACON

When I walked into the hospital room, I saw a lanky man in his hospital gown, looking much younger than his eighty-six years, struggling with his much smaller wife. He was swearing like a sailor as she tried to calm him down. A nurse efficiently pulled up the bed barriers and put the fall-risk monitor in place.

I knew this man. I had treated him on a previous hospital visit, and I knew his present behavior was quite out of character. As he attempted to climb over the bed rails to escape, he made it clear he wanted two things: (a) to go home, and (b) to know where his doctor was (meaning his primary care physician whom he had been seeing for three decades).

On his prior visit, I had explained that his doctor no longer came to the hospital and that I would be caring for him while he was there. Obviously, that conversation had been long forgotten. But I remembered from our previous interaction that his greatest concern was for his wife, who was battling dementia. He was her safe keeper. He could not leave her at home by herself.

I grabbed his hand in a firm handshake and said, "Mr. Howard, I'm Dr. Pyle. I'm going to be your doctor while you're here in the hospital, and we are going to get you home as soon as possible. If you'd like, we can let your wife stay here with you."

Abracadabra! My words worked like magic. He calmed down instantly. Then, as we visited, sweet Mrs. Howard began taking notes in her indecipherable handwriting, just as she had done during the previous hospital visit. She asked me to repeat my name and her husband's diagnosis. She asked for the name of his doctor—the one he had been seeing for thirty years. Coping mechanisms are comforting, and writing was one of Mrs. Howard's.

Previously, Mr. Howard had been admitted because of a heart attack. His hospital stay had been uneventful until three days after admission when he became confused and combative. We searched for the cause. This change of mental status in the elderly can occur due to medication changes, infection, and even just the change to an unfamiliar and therefore frightening location. During his previous stay, he had developed a urinary tract infection (UTI) unrelated to his heart attack but the underlying cause of his confusion. A UTI was also the reason for his current admission.

Medically, his temporary confusion is known as delirium. But delirium for something as minimal as a UTI rarely occurs in a healthy brain. Something else was going on.

I knew Mr. Howard had early dementia from prior medical

records from his doctor. Even so, he was the primary caregiver for a wife with more advanced dementia. This is a common thread woven together by decades of marriage—one spouse caring for another attempting to remain at home as long as possible.

When some patients face the flurry of activity and emotions associated with an unexpected hospitalization, it can feel like losing control. The patient and those who live with them, especially spouses, wonder, *What do we do now? We have not prepared for this. How do we keep our freedom?*[1] Loved ones contemplate the same things, including, *How do we keep* our *freedom when Mom or Dad or both need more care?*

We experience life with the illusion of control. When our journey takes a turn and that illusion is revealed, it is natural to cling to what vestige remains. Control is impossible because there are too many external variables. Mr. Howard struggled mightily because he had enough awareness to know that he was not acting normally, which made him feel like he was losing control. Allowing him to make the decision whether his wife stayed gave him the sense of autonomy he sought. Even when you're in a foreign and confusing situation, you, too, can maintain autonomy for as long as possible—if you have a plan in place.

Looking for a Map

As I walk the halls of my hospital, I pass many who wear the confused look of travelers in a strange land. They are like immigrants, refugees, or tourists on a terrible trip, shuffling papers as they walk along the sterile corridors, reading each sign as they pass. They are obviously lost.

The only directional sign they remember is to take the elevator to a particular floor. This common feature in most hospitals leads to patient rooms. It often becomes a place where families like theirs squeeze into the small space, all anxious to reach their destination.

I can tell they are overwhelmed, afraid, and unsure about how things work and where things are, as Mr. and Mrs. Howard were. I try to make eye contact. I smile and send up silent prayers for comfort. I point and say, "Turn left, then left again, then right, and you'll see the elevators." If I have time, I walk them to their destination. I understand them. I have *been* them.

In a doctor's office or in the emergency department (ED), these visitors have recently watched a family member's passport get stamped "Disease A" and have been directed into the bowels of the hospital for admission. They are ill prepared for the sights, sounds, smells, and inner workings of a hospital.

As they attempt to navigate the physical structure of this unfamiliar new world, their minds are racing with a thousand questions: *What now? Who should we call? What did that nurse say? Who will be the doctor? When will I see my spouse/child/mother/father/friend? How are we going to pay for this? Where is that elevator?*

Meanwhile, while being transported from one strange place to another, the prone patient watches ceiling tiles fly by and listens to nurses talk about their day. He or she is also full of questions: *When will I see my family again? Was that a doctor or a nurse? When can I get something for my pain? Have these nurses forgotten that I can hear them? Am I completely lost in this foreign land? Oh, here's the elevator; I remember them telling my family about the elevator. I hope they see the directional sign. Should I ask these nurses?*

The Stripping Effect

Most people do not get to see a doctor they recognize when a medical crisis erupts. Instead, they show up at an unfamiliar hospital, and what has been described as a "stripping process" begins. In 1975, Dr. Hans Mauksch applied this sociological principle to hospital settings. He noted how patients are almost always forced to endure a bit of waiting. In fact, "waiting in itself can be an expression of power by the institution which makes you wait . . . and is the price you pay for the privilege of obtaining health services."[2]

Along with surrendering to a slow-moving clock, you soon surrender your belongings, your medicines, and your clothing, that last bastion of dignity. Now stripped, both figuratively and literally, you wait some more for your doctor, only to discover that it will not be *your* physician you will be seeing. You will see a doctor you have never seen before. After a brisk introduction, this strange doctor will launch into a barrage of questions.

Mauksch noted, "This climate of dependence on staff and on the institution drains the patient's sense of uniqueness and of human worth."[3] And that can hurt. Soon you are wondering, *Why am I being asked about difficulty with urination when my problem has nothing to do with my bladder?* You fight frustration and cross your fingers that this new doctor knows what he or she is doing.

For Mr. and Mrs. Howard, memory loss resulted in "new doctors" with each visit to the hospital. If possible, it's important for family and caregivers to be present during this transition of care. But if not, being prepared for a transition can relieve some of the unfamiliarity inherent in the stripping effect.

If you have family members like Mr. and Mrs. Howard, create a medical record folder they can bring with them whenever they receive medical care. It is easier to remember to bring a folder than to remember a detailed medical history. It would also be helpful for them always to bring along blank paper and a pen. Equip them to share and gather information easily whenever you cannot be present.

Transitions of Care

I have worked as an internal medicine doctor since 1989, in hospital-based settings for most of my career. The hospitalist model of care freed up primary care physicians (PCPs) from having to make hospital visits, so they could see more patients in their practices and be available for those needing urgent appointments. These days, seldom do we see the busy PCPs visiting patients at the hospital due to time constraints.

It seemed to be a win-win, unless you expected your PCP to visit you in the hospital before and after their office hours as they once had. In those cases, the new arrangement proved to be confusing, frustrating, and scary. The stripping effect was amplified. Patients can feel they have also been stripped of their trusted physicians.

For the hospitalist model to work most effectively, healthcare providers, both in and out of the hospital setting, must communicate efficiently. The development of electronic health records (EHR) has made this sharing of information possible. There are still times, however, when systems do not "talk" properly to one another.

Failure of communication is the most common medical error.[4] Records can be sent instantly, but that does not mean they always are. That's why, across the healthcare sector, developers are creating systems that can be used across providers and organizations to share information and therefore provide better care.

In the event of hospitalization, PCPs are now able to provide a patient's EHR, including ongoing lists of medical diagnoses, surgical histories, medications, personal notes, details, and more. This information in the electronic health record gives the hospitalist a broad framework of the patient's medical history. This is valuable during stressful times when patients and families are inclined to forget important details. Mr. Howard had been in our hospital previously and therefore his medical record was easily accessible from his previous visit. But his PCP used a different EHR, and I did not have access to those records until the PCP's office opened.

To overcome this potential difficulty between clinical visits, ask for printed copies of all new medical records after each visit to your doctor. Patients have easy access to their health records; all you have to do is ask. But you must give permission for family members, caregivers, or anyone else to obtain medical records. This is generally done when checking into any clinical facility.

Also, some larger medical practices and most hospitals have patient portals where you can access your medical records online. Ask if this is available at your clinical care site. I would recommend printing these to keep in a file at home.

Some patients are reluctant to provide access to their medical records even to family members. I find that as the more patients age, the more private they become with their health records. This may be a result of fears associated with loss of autonomy.

This underscores the importance of planning in advance for times like Mr. Howard's family was facing. It is *always* better to have discussions about these issues when the patient is not in crisis. That leaves room to develop a safe plan of care that creates autonomy and allows one or more trusted family members to participate in the patient's health journey.

Be proactive in these steps of shared decision-making.

Keep copies of the records to help you become the best healthcare advocate for yourself or someone else in the following locations:

- Patient's home, in an easily retrievable location
- A fireproof safe box
- Car, in the event of an emergency
- Healthcare proxy or power of attorney's home (roles will be defined in later chapters)
- Caregiver's or family's home
- If traveling, carry a copy with you or be able to access if digital

While many of these records may transfer seamlessly, it is always best to hand the clinician a physical copy that they can scan quickly in the event of an emergency.

The transfer process repeats in reverse when the hospitalist transfers care of the patient back to their PCP. Before they're discharged, patients are given a summary of their hospital stay diagnoses and what's known as a *medication reconciliation* (often referred to as a "med rec"). This document is a record of all medications taken *prior* to a hospital stay, which ones are to be continued *after* the hospital stay, and which new ones were added *during* the hospital stay.

It's always better that the patient has a family member or caregiver present at the time of the discharge process. It is helpful to have a second set of ears to hear the instructions. This is especially important to prevent taking medications that might have been stopped during the hospital stay.

Patients should always request from the discharging doctor that a copy of their detailed *medical discharge summary* be sent to their

PCP and additional care providers. For example, a cancer patient would have it sent to their PCP and their oncologist, a cancer specialist. This record describes the hospital visit in more detail than what the patient receives at discharge. It may not be available for up to a week following discharge. Patients or those who have been given permission by the patient can obtain the document from their PCP.

If all this sounds overwhelming, that's understandable. But remember knowledge is power, and the more you know, the easier things will be.

The Power of Knowledge

A map or GPS provides comfort and knowledge when you're traveling in foreign lands. In the foreign land of a hospital, knowledge will also bring you comfort. Knowledge gives power. Knowledge gives dignity. Knowledge gives peace.

For patients and caregivers, roles may change at any given time—as they did with Mr. and Mrs. Howard. Mrs. Howard was trying her best to understand by writing notes. Though her notes were indecipherable, I encouraged her to continue because it brought her comfort and made her feel she was caring for her husband as he had cared for her.

In the foreign land of a hospital, knowledge will also bring you comfort. Knowledge gives power. Knowledge gives dignity. Knowledge gives peace.

I'd encourage the same impulse in you as well. Expand your knowledge and collect information as you go. To help you along the way, I want to give you a road map of what you should know if you enter the healthcare system. Every country has a unique healthcare system and strategies will change; however, the principles of these recommendations are applicable to most systems. These are my suggestions for patients and those who care for them to prepare for an unexpected hospital stay.

WHAT TO KNOW

- **Know how your healthcare system works.** If you call for an ambulance, where would you be taken? If you live in a country that does not have a centralized call system, what would you do if you had an emergency? Do you have options for healthcare that you should be choosing now? For example, in the United States, your options are contained within an insurance system. Do you have traditional insurance, Medicare, or are you part of a closed healthcare system such as a health maintenance organization (HMO)? Or do you still need to choose? Take the time now to understand the healthcare choices you have, regardless of age or health status. If you don't have choices, learn how to make the most of the healthcare system available to you by asking to speak to a caseworker within your system.
- **Know the local hospitals.** Most hospitals measure, monitor, and publicize how quickly they deliver care. It is wise to know the track records of the facilities in your area. Consider online resources to check the quality of clinical facilities near you.

- Medicare, www.medicare.gov, under the "Providers and Services" tab
- *U.S. News & World Report*, www.usnews.com, under the "Health" section
- Leapfrog Hospital Safety Grade, www.hospitalsafetygrade.org

Clinical locations such as hospitals, skilled nursing facilities, and hospices are rated with various parameters on these websites. The Medicare website also gives accreditation to qualifying facilities. Many facilities, especially hospices, are not accredited. I would consider this as you make choices. Likewise, clinical providers are rated based upon specialty and quality.[5]

- **Know your doctor's approach**. Discuss with your primary care physician whether he or she still "makes rounds" (visits hospitalized patients). If not (most likely he or she does not), ask his or her opinion on the quality of the hospitalists or physician groups at area hospitals.
- **Know your wishes.** Keep a copy of specific medical orders such as Do Not Resuscitate or Do Not Intubate. We will talk much more about advance care plans (ACP) in coming chapters, but you can refer to Resource B: Guide to Documents and Advance Planning at the back of the book for descriptions of different types of planning tools and specific order sets that transfer with you between clinical locations.
- **Know your plan.** Again, we'll review more in coming chapters about developing an acute illness plan, but

whatever plan you have, make sure to have it accessible. This includes an accurate list of medications, current doctors' names, prior surgeries and illnesses, medical diagnoses, emergency contacts, and your ACP, which I hope you will have developed by the time you finish this book or shortly thereafter.

- **Know your companions.** When the patient is in the hospital, I highly recommend a family member or other health advocate stay with the patient at night. This is especially true for the elderly, those who are at risk for falls, and those with a serious or terminal illness. Medication error is more likely to occur at night[6] and between the hours of 7 and 8 a.m. and 7 and 8 p.m.[7] As part of your plan, you can decide who your hospital companion will be ahead of time, and make sure to include that person on your list of emergency contacts.
- **Know what to bring.** Create a medical "waiting bag." This bag can include anything that would help you pass the time if you or a family member were to spend an excessive amount of time waiting for an assessment. This could include provisions of comfort such as a small travel blanket and travel pillow. For spiritual comfort, include a Bible and perhaps a devotional guide. Bring a notebook and pen so you can write your questions and add notes as the doctor or nurse gives you information.
- **Know how to stay comfortable**. Keep hand sanitizer, water bottles, snacks, and at least a twenty-four-hour supply of your routine medications in your bag. If you

are the patient, hospitalists will want to look at each of the medications and dosages you are taking. If you are admitted, they will most likely *not* want you to take your own medication. This helps to prevent duplication of medication doses. Family members should bring their medications to prevent missing a dose if they stay as well. Emergency departments and hospitals are often cold and uncomfortable. A blanket or pillow from home can make a big difference.

- **Know how to update others.** Most emergency departments are busy and allow only one or two family members or friends to be with a patient at any given time. Have a plan in place to receive and relay information to other loved ones reliably. (We'll talk about building a call tree later.)
- **Know you may move.** If a hospital physician recommends a transfer to another medical facility, realize this is in the best interest of the patient. Specific laws guide interfacility transfers in the United States as well as other healthcare delivery systems. The primary criterion is a patient's unmet need at the current hospital can be met at the receiving facility.
- **Know the schedule.** After you're admitted to a hospital, inquire when the hospitalist on duty makes rounds so family members may be present for exams or consultations. Ask for a window of time if the clinician is reluctant to give a precise time.
- **Know the right questions.** Prepare a list of questions in

advance and take notes during the hospital stay to help you remember. (Mrs. Howard wisely took notes, but her dementia prevented her from understanding why she took them.) In the previous chapter, we explored questions to ask about a diagnosis. Here are a few more to ask in the hospital or doctor's office before a test, procedure, or treatment is administered.

  - Do I really need this test, procedure, or treatment?
  - Will doing this test change the management of my care?
  - What are the risks of this test, procedure, or treatment?
  - Are there alternative options?
  - What are the potential outcomes if I choose not to do this procedure or treatment?[8]

- **Know your rights.** You have the right to be treated with dignity and respect, to have your questions answered, and to say no to a test, procedure, or treatment. You have the right to ask for a second opinion. You have the right to make a formal complaint to the hospital's administration. These and other rights are communicated through the Patients' Bill of Rights, which is available on the federal government's website.[9] Additional rights are added periodically, and these additions can be found on the website www.medicare.gov. The Patient Advocate Foundation at www.patientadvocate.org provides educational resources on your rights as patients and loved ones.[10]

The Local Guides

When in a foreign land, it is helpful to know there are locals to guide you. This is especially true when the land is the intensive care unit (ICU). Some larger facilities not only have hospitalists on staff, but physicians known as *intensivists.* These specialists typically care for critically ill patients in ICUs. In an open ICU, a more general hospitalist may also care for patients. In a closed ICU, patients will be seen only by the intensivist, with the hospitalist resuming care for the patient when he or she moves to a regular hospital room. In both cases, the first set of rounds is generally made early in the morning.

Nurses will hurry in and out of patient rooms all hours of the day and night, plugging and unplugging tubes, injecting medicines, and caring for a patient even as they listen attentively to the beeps and sounds coming from the room next door. As a group, ICU nurses tend to be extremely smart and highly driven. They routinely see the worst of patient tragedies.

In my experience, working in such conditions tends to create nurses with either a thick, self-protective shell or nurses with profound faith. Patients and families must quickly determine which type of nurse is caring for them. This is important to do, because your ICU nurse will often act as your *interpreter* when you do not understand medical jargon. They are *strength bearers* in times of weakness, *guides* during moments of indecision, and *encouragers* in periods of despair. They are unsung heroes. By building a relationship with their caregivers in the hospital or ICU, patients and families can enhance their experience even if an illness is quite serious.

You may find yourself with a nurse who seems to bear a self-protective shell and lack compassion, empathy, and wisdom. In that case, begin with kindness. *How are you? We are so grateful for your care. Have you been a nurse a long time? What do you like about your job? Do you have a family?* It is surprising how quickly walls drop after simple acts of unexpected kindness.

Then humanize your loved one, the patient. Pictures, stories, and family memories help clinicians feel vested in unique ways to care for the patient before them. It is simple psychology but highly effective. Finally, if neither of these strategies works, it is your right to ask for another nurse.

I won't forget what I witnessed working in one tiny ICU, ten beds in all, in a small hospital in a small town. I could tell this place was special the moment I entered. Each morning I watched Carol, the unit's manager, go from room to room greeting patients and inquiring about their night. Carol had a special gift—a compassion that transcended sympathy. She had empathy in spades.

This empathy was grounded in her deep faith, and as a pastor's wife, she shared it willingly with those around her. She had the ability not only to care for a patient's suffering but also to share in it. Her leadership was infectious, and she created a culture of caring compassion among the staff in this little ICU.

However, empathy without excellence in medical knowledge and quality care is much like a two-legged stool, not safe to sit upon. This small ICU not only had Carol, but it also had Dr. Po, the smartest doctor I have ever met. Each morning, Dr. Po worked side by side with his dedicated nursing staff, continually sharing his immense medical knowledge.

Though I have been trained in some of the largest, most advanced ICUs in the world, it was in this ICU that I learned my greatest lessons, the greatest of which was the power of *hope* that can be transmitted through caring medical professionals. They are your guides in what can be a baffling foreign land.

Though you might not have Carol in the ICU, hope can still exist and may be found in others. Many night-shift nurses have a rare ability to exude peace as the ICU settles down after a frantic day. These night angels are sources of information for patients and families who need a deeper understanding of the day's events. And all nurses and intensivists can provide guidance that helps you determine a way forward, whatever life may bring outside the hospital.

For those admitted to the hospital, I often recommend loved ones bring a photo of the patient before they were sick to keep at the bedside (whether or not they are in the ICU). This simple act of revealing a life that existed before an illness helps clinicians see past the human life they are interacting with in the moment. It is a *humanizer*. Finding that human connection in the hospital can be a light in the darkness, something to hold on to in a healthcare system that feels so foreign.

QUESTIONS FOR THE ICU

No matter what time you or your loved one arrives in the ICU, consider asking the following questions to map your way forward in intensive care.

- Doctor, will you be the only doctor on my/his/her case, or will there be others?
- What time do you make rounds, and what time would be

best to receive an update? For loved ones: If visiting hours do not coincide with the time you are making rounds, may we schedule time with you to discuss the care of our loved one?

- Is a family member or caregiver allowed to stay with the patient overnight?
- If there are any significant changes, will you or your nurse give a prompt update? For loved ones: Does your nurse have our cell number(s) for updates? When should we expect to hear from you?
- If we have questions between visiting hours or rounds, what is the best way to communicate those?
- If you are given two options for treatment: If this were your family member, what would you do?
- Are there any questions we have not asked, but should ask?

The Path Through Fear

My friend, can we pause for a moment? While I write, I think of you and pray for you. Are you the patient reading all this information and wondering what lies ahead? Are you feeling fearful and paralyzed by the unknown? Fear is one of the many emotions people experience in this foreign land.

Fear's primary function is to signal us to the threat of danger and trigger an appropriate protective response. Fear is experienced in the mind, yet the body has a strong physical reaction. Mr. Howard, the patient I told you about at the beginning of this chapter, had a violent reaction.

Medically, fear can affect the part of the brain that processes judgment and rational thinking. A sense of dread and anxiety can replace logic and can lead to panic.

In serious medical situations, fear of the unknown can make us feel lost. Yet with planning and knowledge, preparation and human connection, we can lessen the sting of the fears that are certain to arise.

By the time of Mr. Howard's discharge, he had returned to his functional baseline mental status, which was kind and thoughtful. I discussed with him and his wife a thorough discharge plan. I encouraged them to begin formulating with their children a plan for when they would no longer be able to live at home alone.

This subject was upsetting to Mrs. Howard. I could feel her fear. Even the innocuous thought of having home health provide occasional help was upsetting to her. With Mr. Howard's permission, I also spoke with the couple's daughter. I alerted her to the life and health issues that were looming and that needed to be addressed sooner rather than later.

If you find yourself in this circumstance, it is vital to have a plan in place. Families must come together and formulate a plan of care when both parents are not in the hospital and not under undue stress. Both parents should engage in this process early and often. This will help give them a sense of autonomy in a world where it can feel like their freedom is rapidly slipping away.

That afternoon, I was getting on the elevator as Mr. Howard was exiting in a wheelchair, pushed by one of the many wonderful hospital volunteers. Mrs. Howard followed closely behind. I gave them each a hug and was thankful to hear Mr. Howard say, "Thank you, Doctor, for your care. Our daughter came to visit and is giving us a ride home. Isn't that great?"

I reflect on this moment with a smile now and think they seemed a lot less lost than they had the first time they took that elevator. With a map and a plan in hand, they have a way forward, all the way home.

> *But grow in the grace and knowledge of*
> *our Lord and Savior Jesus Christ.*
> *To him be the glory both now and forever. Amen.*
> 2 PETER 3:18

four

DIMINISHING CHAOS

Death is as near to the young as to the old; here is all the difference: death stands behind the young man's back, before the old man's face.

THOMAS ADAMS

Though I had been trained in one of the nation's largest and most renowned hospital systems, my first position was in a smaller hospital in South Carolina that served a beachside community that swelled and shrank depending on the season.

Every fall, big flocks of retired "snowbirds" descended upon us. These travelers fled the harsh winters of New England and Canada and made local hotel owners grateful to turn on their No Vacancy signs. In spring and summer, the town played host to countless golfers and vacationing families.

Every step of my medical training and practicing medicine brought fresh challenges and responsibilities. The most difficult transition was from medical resident to employed physician. I no longer had a resident, fellow, or attending physician to back me up in the event of a critical case. I *was* the backup. What's more, our hospital had very few specialists at the time, which was unnerving. I felt the full weight of the doctor's role for the first time.

Thankfully, I realized the old medical adage is true: if you listen to your patients long enough, they will tell you what their diagnosis is. With the right questions and active listening, the repetitive nature of my training kicked in. I tapped into the layers of memories from my medical education, and those would result in a correct diagnosis and proper treatment regimen. I came to enjoy the feel and work pace of a hospital and the ratio of routine to unexpected cases.

Nevertheless, medicine is still medicine, and not every outcome is good. Sometimes you have the weighty responsibility of sharing a difficult diagnosis. It is hard enough watching a sixty-six-year-old husband weep when he realizes that, barring a miracle, his wife does not have much time left. It is even more gut-wrenching when tragedy strikes the young.

The Fragility of Life

I was working the night shift when I received a call from the emergency department: "I'm going to need you to come down to see a patient. It's a tough one."

"Tough" was putting it mildly. Two young newlyweds had come to our resort town, the words "Just Married!" scrawled in big letters across the back window of their car. For fun, they had attended one of the many theaters in our area. A few of these theaters thrilled guests with elaborate, grandiose shows. This couple chose one that featured skilled riders on horseback performing acrobatics as they raced around the ring. Meanwhile, acrobatics continued high in the theater in tandem with those on the ground. It was a favorite of both locals and visitors.

Soon after entering the theater, the young husband complained of shortness of breath. When his condition worsened, someone called 911. Before an emergency crew could arrive, the man collapsed, his lips turning blue. It was determined later that dander from the horses in the show had triggered a severe allergic reaction.

A crowd gathered around the collapsed man, unsure of what to do until the ambulance arrived. The frantic wife knelt by his head, calling his name. The scene was chaotic, the sense of panic increasing with each passing moment.

The new bride, whom I later learned was pregnant, could only stand by helplessly as paramedics worked feverishly to get an airway into her husband's swollen windpipe. As the ambulance doors closed, she saw them administering cardiopulmonary resuscitation (CPR).

The emergency medical technicians could not afford to be distracted, so the bride was not allowed to ride in the ambulance. I later spoke to the kind theater manager, who described the events and had driven her to the hospital. I can only imagine her desire to keep seeing the ambulance lights in the distance, an invisible tether to her groom. He was placed immediately on life support upon arrival to the emergency department. His scared, solitary wife was ushered into a room to wait.

As I hung up the phone and headed downstairs, my heart broke for this young couple. Tragedy leaves an indelible imprint. We don't believe it will happen to us, until it does. My strength—and, I suppose, my weakness—is my ability to feel deeply the pain of patients and families who are suffering. I needed to take care of him, but I also wanted to comfort her.

In the ED, I consulted again with the staff who were attending to this young man. They were visibly shaken by the tragedy unfolding in their midst.

"Has he had any sedation?" I asked.

"No. Nothing, not even in transport."

This was not good news. The only movement I witnessed was the patient's chest rising and falling with each artificially supplied breath. He was not struggling against the ventilator. His pupils were fixed and dilated, and no reflexes were noted.

As I continued my exam, I began processing internally the gravity of the situation. I thought about the waiting bride and what I would say to her. I asked myself the same questions that she must have thought: *How can this be happening? Is this real?*

I completed the orders to get him transferred to the ICU and took a deep breath before entering the tiny consultation room. It contained two chairs and a couch, sterile and cold. The only warmth was a picture of the beach that hung somewhat crookedly in its artificial wood frame.

A young woman was sitting on the end of the couch, her knees drawn tightly to her chest. She looked up expectantly, tears streaming down her face.

"Is he okay? Is he okay?" she asked, searching my face for any hint of good news.

I sat down next to her and held her hands, hoping my eyes did not convey my deep concern.

I cleared my throat before speaking. "My name is Dr. Pyle, and I will be taking care of your husband. He has had an allergic reaction called anaphylaxis. We're concerned that his brain did not receive enough oxygen, and therefore, he's on life support . . . but he's not waking up. We're going to bring him to the ICU and hope that we see some change over the next twenty-four hours."

"But . . . but, he *will* wake up, right?" she asked plaintively.

"It's possible, yet it's too early to tell," I said quietly. "We can hope things will change. Would you like me to call his family, or would you?"

She hugged her knees tighter and began to sob uncontrollably. I put my arms around her the way a mother hugs a scared child. My daughters were not much younger than she was. As I did, she melted into me.

Afterward, I made a call to his parents and said the words no mother or father wants to hear: "Come now."

Unfortunately, I could not deliver good news that evening, or the next day, or the day after that. A neurologist grimly confirmed our worst fears. Because of a prolonged lack of oxygen to the young husband's brain during his allergic episode, he now met the clinical criteria for brain death.

Brain death *is* death, but it is much harder for loved ones to process. Unlike cardiovascular death, where a patient's body quickly grows cold, with brain death, the body remains warm for an extended period as machines work to replicate life. (Resource C describes what you need to know about brain death criteria.)

Almost from the beginning, the new bride's face was etched with deep grief. She seemed to know her husband was gone. As assorted family members arrived during the next twenty-four hours, this brave young woman helped them understand as well.

Though she was still too early in her pregnancy to have a baby bump, I noticed the way she kept touching her stomach as if cradling the memory, and the legacy, of a deep love cut short.

The young bride quickly understood the clinical criteria for brain death. She also understood its finality. Her heart was shattered, yet she never rushed any of her husband's loved ones through their questions, and when she needed help, she asked us to help her explain.

While it was her decision to remove life support, she relied upon his family's support. Eventually she shared with them that on his driver's license application, this young husband had checked the box that read, "Yes, I would like to donate my organs."

I do not know if this young man had a will or a life insurance policy, but he had prepared at least this much for death. If his life ended prematurely, he had made it clear that he wanted to give life to others. His ending plan was simple. He chose life.

The Plan Everyone Needs

In general, we are planners by nature. We plan weddings, children, birthdays, anniversaries, trips, sizing homes up and down, and finally for retirement. Most people live by their planners, calendars, or some such bearer of a life plan. A plan is needed just as much in the world of healthcare crises, where tragedies unfold in diseases that slowly deteriorate the body but not the mind, or diseases that slowly cloud the mind until thoughts can't escape.

This type of plan is called an advance care plan, or ACP. An ACP speaks for you if you are unable to speak for yourself due to a medical condition. It is also a vehicle to express your faith, your legacy, and your final wishes, such as becoming an organ donor.

If you are facing a life-changing health event and your journey as a patient is just beginning, you may feel uncomfortable bringing up the topic of an ACP. You are just beginning the battle and have plenty of fight in you. An ACP may seem like surrendering or being too pessimistic.

But having and fully understanding an ACP may be one of the greatest gifts you can give to those who love you. I know it must be difficult for you to think of such matters when you carry so much hope and faith. It may seem counterintuitive, but it is not.

Through all my patient experiences and brushes with my own mortality, I've recognized that death may arrive on any day and in any way. Having an ACP in place equips you for the unexpected, allowing the more valuable aspects of living and dying to be shared with the ones you love.

I chose to complete an ACP because I didn't want to miss a single day of anticipating heaven. I didn't want to be Scarlett O'Hara from *Gone with the Wind*, who said petulantly, "I can't think about that right now. If I do, I'll go crazy. I'll think about it tomorrow."[1]

If you are facing death, you do think about tomorrow. You have gained new perspective, and you treasure each of your tomorrows while you fully live your todays. Yet, like many, you may wonder, *How many tomorrows will I be given, and what will they bring?*

Beginning with an ending plan allows you and your family to live each tomorrow focused on the lovely things in life. Manage what requires management now. You and your family will want your ending tomorrows to be filled with peace, joy, love, and worship, rather than fretful or panicky decision-making.

The Gold Standard

The truth is, if you don't plan now for the unexpected, some level of chaos will inevitably ensue. Chaos during a medical crisis can break hearts, create division among family members, detract from the patient's needs—and is *entirely avoidable* with a proper plan.

An ACP is the gold standard for addressing all aspects of care, not only near the end of life but in any illness when a patient is incapable of making decisions for him or herself. Examples of the latter would be a patient in a coma from medical causes or traumatic brain injuries, severe dementia, or a persistent vegetative state. These events can occur without warning. They can also occur at the end of a protracted illness. Life does not discriminate on when they occur.

It is never too early or too late to complete an ACP. ACPs encompass the preparation of legal documents. They can also guide discussions with family members and physicians about what the future may hold for the expected and unexpected. The ACP is a tool to help alleviate concerns related to finances, family matters, spiritual questions, and other issues that trouble seriously ill or dying patients and their families.[2]

An ACP sometimes incorporates previously communicated wishes (and/or documents) created under the legal transactional approach, such as a living will or healthcare power of attorney. (For more on the descriptions for planning tools, refer to Resource B at the back of this book.) The ACP is meant to be reviewed annually or whenever there are significant changes in one's medical condition.

The benefits of ACPs for individuals, families, and society at large are well documented.[3] These include the following:

- Higher rates of your wishes being fulfilled (for example, through a living will, healthcare power of attorney, or combined advance directives)
- Increased likelihood that clinicians and families will understand and comply with a patient's wishes

- A reduction in hospitalization at the end of life
- The receipt of less intensive treatments at the end of life
- Increase of hospice services
- Increased likelihood that a patient will die in his or her preferred place
- Higher satisfaction with the quality of care
- Better family preparation on what to expect during the dying process
- Lower risk of stress, anxiety, and depression in surviving relatives of deceased persons
- Greater receptivity to end-of-life discussions by patients and families
- Reduced cost of end-of-life care without increasing mortality[4]

That is quite a list of benefits! Even so, few people complete an ACP, and even fewer fully understand its purpose when they are in a time of need. I urge you, therefore, to look through the next chapters carefully, and ideally with family members young and old. It begins with an advocate—and that can be you.

Death Personified

It is difficult to consider an ending without also having hope for a beginning. I imagine you have visualized Death as the grim reaper, scythe in hand, eyes covered in darkness from his hooded cloak. We envision Death's sting as the scythe moves through the air, and we flinch at the thought of metal striking flesh. Yet God's Word reveals the truth about this Death who invades our nightmares:

> Yea, though I walk through the valley of the shadow of death,
> I will fear no evil;
> For You are with me;
> Your rod and Your staff, they comfort me. (Psalm 23:4)

The Christian believer, through faith in Jesus Christ, experiences only the *shadow of death*. We can anticipate heaven by experiencing life with the understanding that the death we have known prior to salvation exists only as a mere shadow of a future that is no longer ours. If we choose to personify Death, we can envision the friend who walks us into the loving arms of our Savior. Perspective is everything as you face the end of life.

Life from Death

Years after the death of the young husband, I think about his bride and their child, who would now be an adult. I do not know what happened to them, but I know this: the mother can proudly tell her son or daughter, "Your father was a hero. As a young man, he made a commitment that if tragic circumstances ever took his life, he would, in death, give life. And he did."

This simple act of checking a box on a government form is small in the scheme of the planning we do during life. Yet it meant the world to his bride and those whose lives were changed because of his sacrifice. Though she no longer had him in life, in death she honored his wish to donate his organs and help others. Her family's heartache could at least give hope to one or more families. The young husband had planned in the event of a tragedy. This plan helped create order in chaos. As we continue, we'll explore in more detail the possibilities of an advance care plan, and the order and peace it could create for you and your loved ones when the unexpected happens.

> *I will both lie down in peace, and sleep; For you alone, O Lord, make me dwell in safety.*
>
> PSALM 4:8

five

A BARGAIN AND A TREASURE

Once you know that catastrophe dwells next door and can strike anyone at any time, you interpret reality differently.

RONNIE JANOFF-BULMAN

Lizzy was the only girl and the youngest. Her two older brothers adored their much younger sister. She was also the apple of her father's eye. Her recollection of her younger years were bedtime stories "told from scratch" and Saturday pancakes with chocolate chips that her father made for the whole family. She would see him wink as she delighted in the smiley-faced pancakes he shaped just for her.

As the years passed, father and daughter kept this special bond. She would do anything to be around him, even go to the flea market on Saturday mornings after pancakes, which he loved to do. When she asked what he was hoping to find, he replied, "I'm just looking for some treasure that someone might not have wanted."

As her brothers went to college, she still called him Daddy. They all looked forward to those rare weekends when they could be together again. But when it came time for her to leave for school, her heart was torn between the world she knew and the world she was about to enter. Her mom told her years later that her daddy had buried his head in her shoulder, weeping, as their daughter turned the corner to go to her dorm. Lizzy wished she would have known.

During her sophomore year in college, she received *the* call from her brother. He said, "Sis, I need you to be calm, but they just took Dad to the hospital. Aunt Sharon called, and they think he had a stroke. You need to tell your roommate to notify the school and head home. We will meet you there." She doesn't remember the ride home, but she does remember the words "massive stroke" as the doctor spoke.

Days of not knowing if he would survive turned to weeks and then months of care at the hospital and a rehabilitation facility. Even though he was unable to move one side of his body, he seemed to have hope that defied explanation. She wanted to hope with him, but reality grounded her steps. She realized that, barring a bona fide miracle, her father would never walk again, drive again, or leave the care of nurses. Their family would never be the same.

What she did not know was how the next hard months would become an unexpected gift. Her incapacitated father would still be the Daddy she had always known. Lizzy and her family moved her ailing father to a nearby nursing home that could provide the care and rehabilitation services he needed. She withdrew from school to be close.

The stroke had stripped him of his physical capacities, but the parts of him that made her love him remained the same. Father and daughter began to enjoy laughter over silly things and marvel at memories of beautiful times. Their special relationship grew even in this darkest hour. She felt like she had time to learn the "why" and the "how" he had become the man he was.

A few things kept this daddy going, kept him trying, and kept him alive. One was his hope. He hoped he might one day dance with his daughter at her wedding. His greater motivation, however, was that he might have more time to show each of his children and his wife how great his love was for them.

Providentially, a few months prior to his stroke, he had spent time thinking about and planning for a scenario just like this one. He had discovered an ACP document called the Five Wishes.[1] He was an attorney and knew its value even if its price tag was "less than one of those fancy cups of coffee he wouldn't be caught drinking."

When Lizzy, my friend, gets to this part of her family's story, I can always hear the smile in her voice. She quips, "Daddy always loved a good bargain, and I think he was prouder of the bargain he got than he was of the fact that he had completed the document!"

Like many of us, this father had no warning about the events he would soon be facing. Yet by completing the Five Wishes and sharing it with his children, he continued to be Daddy to them. He was loving them in a way not even he could have fathomed.

The family took the time in those final months to discuss his wishes, and as they did, he affirmed the value of the exercise, not how little it cost. Through this process, father and daughter learned more about each other. Sometimes they wept together, while other times they laughed hysterically.

This daddy gave one of the best gifts a parent can give a child—time. During those long conversations, he also gave other gifts: expressions of faith, peace of mind, and good memories.

A Disguised Treasure

I smile when I think of this daddy. Who doesn't like a bargain? We all do! Oftentimes with bargain shopping, however, we end up accepting things of lesser quality, or we settle for items that are slightly damaged.

The Five Wishes is *not* that kind of bargain. It is more like a treasure disguised as a bargain. It has been described as "the ACP with heart and soul." The website www.fivewishes.org gives options for a digital or paper version. The digital version is safely stored and can be changed over time. It is available in over thirty languages, including braille.

Imagine: for the cost of a latte or a totally forgettable fast-food meal, you can buy that which becomes priceless. Time spent thinking about such important matters and sharing them with others is time well spent. It is good for all concerned.

An ACP document is comprehensive in scope (covering personal, spiritual, medical, and legal issues). It includes a living will, but also includes other necessary documents. It must be easily understood and meet the legal requirements of your state or country. If a legal document is not required where you live, an ACP still provides a framework to guide decisions in the event you are no longer able to communicate your decisions.

In the United States, the National Hospice and Palliative Care Association provides resources for alternatives to the Five Wishes on the website www.caringinfo.org. This website also has a list of companies that provide video and digital versions of an ACP. I personally use and prefer the Five Wishes for its thoroughness and affordability and will use it in this book as our gold standard. (For transparency, I do not receive any fees for this recommendation.)

Regardless of which ACP you and your family choose, it may be an uncomfortable topic to bring up for discussion. But creating an ACP *before* a crisis helps alleviate uncomfortable feelings *during* a crisis. If you as the patient have already received a serious diagnosis, you may need to include this in a family discussion. May I suggest you lead with, "This will help me have more peace, focus on medical treatment, sleep better," and so on. And if you are the one with discomfort answering these questions, give yourself grace. Take some time, and perhaps reread the known benefits of a completed ACP.

Let's Plan Together

I am a mother of five and a grandmother of eight. As I write this, my birthday is approaching. On a previous birthday, I asked my family to complete our Five Wishes together. I expected a varied response, but if using my birthday got buy-in, I had no qualms using it. My children also knew I was writing this book, so I hoped that fact would give me more leverage to tug on their heartstrings. That is how important I believe it is to get this conversation started. My philosophy is "Whatever works!" My encouragement to you is to get started.

If you have already completed an ACP document, grab it and make any needed corrections or clarifications to your end-of-life plan as we go through this material. If you are working with another form of ACP, these general discussions and patient stories will still be of value.

I have cared for thousands of patients in hospital and intensive-care settings over more than three decades. Each patient and their loved ones became my teachers, and I theirs. As you will see in these stories, there will be nuanced differences between the written ACP and the patient experience. Your answers to each question in the ACP are unique. That is okay, because there is not one right answer—only the right one for you.

Ready to start?

These statements are adapted from the Five Wishes document, which I used myself for family.

Wish 1: The Person I Want to Make Healthcare Decisions for Me When I Can't Make Them

This statement regards who your healthcare *proxy* or healthcare *agent* will be. This person may also be called healthcare power of attorney. All three names describe the same role for the person you choose to make healthcare decisions on your behalf in the event you are unable to understand and make informed decisions. I chose my husband, Scott. This was an easy question for me to answer because Scott and I have had so many conversations about these topics. He would know the things I want (and do not want) even if I had not written them down.

If Scott dies before I do, then I have selected my oldest daughter, Amber, as my alternate healthcare proxy. She is practical and logical—an engineer. She would make the difficult decisions. She would also look to her siblings, Brooke, Britney, Dylan, and Christian, for agreement, but would understand that as my proxy, she would make the final decision based upon my wishes.

A few close friends know I want to be cremated and have my ashes spread at a special hidden lake in Colorado. Scott hates this idea and has said that if he is alive, "That's *not* going to happen." Part of me thinks, *I'll be dead at that point, so what's the use in fighting over it?*

But another part of me takes comfort in my secret weapon, my best friend, Kelli. She and I have hiked up to that mountain lake a few times, talking along the way about our families, about life, and our anticipation of heaven and spending eternity together. If anyone will be able to talk Scott into my way of thinking, it's Kelli.

Choosing a healthcare proxy is one of the most important decisions you can make. Typically, it is a spouse or adult child, depending on his or her temperament, personality, maturity, and emotional stability. You may choose someone who is not a family member for this role. If so, I highly recommend that you discuss your reasons with close family members.

For example, it may be that you do not want to "pick" between your children. Or your explanation may be along the lines of, "I didn't want to burden you at a time when I know you will already be grieving. My proxy knows exactly what I want. I would like for you to honor my wishes, and I promise you that I have done this planning because I love you. If or when I cannot speak for myself verbally, my Five Wishes document and my proxy will be saying exactly what I would say if I could."

I should point out the line between "still able to make decisions for myself" and "needing my healthcare proxy to step in" is not always clear. In such gray, fuzzy situations, families often begin making decisions for the patient when in fact he or she could still be making them, perhaps with a little help from clinicians and the designated healthcare proxy.

Lest this possible scenario create tension between you and your family, between family members, or between family and proxy, a good intercessor is needed. You might wish to name a *mediator*, such as a trusted and respected family friend, a pastor, priest, rabbi, or family attorney, to fill this role. Include that detail in your document. Ultimately, a clinician can also advise when there are disagreements between family members and the chosen proxy.

In my document, I describe to whom I have assigned these various roles (healthcare proxy, healthcare proxy alternate, mediator) and why. It is critical the people you select for these various roles feel comfortable accepting them.

You will need to spend time with them reviewing your wishes so there is no misunderstanding *exactly* what you want and do not want. Remember, this is not a popularity contest between your children, siblings, or friends. You are choosing the person(s) you feel can best articulate and implement your wishes.

You may change your mind about your healthcare proxy with age or a change in circumstances. If you *do* make a change, your documents should reflect that change.

I'll Meet You There

As you begin your journey with your advance care plan as a person of faith, do not lose sight of the eternity before you and the heaven you are promised by your Lord and Savior. If you or a loved one is imminently preparing to live in heaven and working on an ACP as you read this, know that each day I pray for you. I may not meet you while I am wearing my earth suit, but when I anticipate heaven, I imagine meeting you and celebrating with you our shared eternity.

What do we know about our heavenly destination?

As believers, we can praise our Father for our eternal home. And as we make choices for ourselves and others, let us remember the grace we are extended and the choice for heaven made possible by Jesus Christ, Prince of Peace, King of kings, Immanuel ("God with us").

What is heaven? Let's look to Scripture for the best descriptions of what we can anticipate.

Heaven Is a Place and a Promise

> *"Let not your heart be troubled; you believe in God, believe also in Me. In My Father's house are many mansions; if it were not so, I would have told you. I go to prepare a place for you."*
>
> JOHN 14:1–2

Because this is true, I *anticipate* dwelling with the One who conquered my death with his life.

Heaven Is in God's Presence and Brings Eternal Pleasures

> *You will show me the path of life; in Your presence is fullness of joy; at Your right hand are pleasures forevermore.*
>
> PSALM 16:11

Because this is true, I *anticipate* the presence of the One who makes my heart sing.

Heaven Is the Home of Perfect Knowledge

> *Now I know in part, but then I shall know just as I also am known.*
>
> 1 CORINTHIANS 13:12

Because this is true, I *anticipate* a time when I will have no unanswered questions.

Heaven Is Prepared for Us by God

As it is written: "Eye has not seen, nor ear heard, nor have entered into the heart of man the things which God has prepared for those who love Him."
1 CORINTHIANS 2:9

Because this is true, I *anticipate* the place where God walks, and the garden humanity was created to inhabit.

I encourage you to read each of these verses and write how you would finish this sentence: *Because this is true, I anticipate . . .* This is one of the ways you will begin to tackle your fears about the end of life on earth.

Dancing in Heaven

Lizzy's father did not walk again, yet he anticipated that heaven would include a Southern dance called "the shag." He never missed an opportunity to point family, friends, and visitors to the heaven he anticipated and the glorious body that would replace "this old sack of clickity, clackity bones."

Oh, glorious day! Heaven is the ultimate destination beyond everything we plan for so carefully on earth. I hope to see you there.

Heaven is the ultimate destination beyond everything we plan for so carefully on earth. I hope to see you there.

> *Our citizenship is in heaven, from which we also eagerly wait for the Savior, the Lord Jesus Christ, who will transform our lowly body that it may be conformed to His glorious body, according to the working by which He is able even to subdue all things to Himself.*
>
> PHILIPPIANS 3:20–21

six

THE HARD HARD CHOICES

Live not for battles won.
Live not for the-end-of-the-song.
Live in the along.
GWENDOLYN BROOKS

The normally jovial Paul was quieter than usual as he loaded my luggage. He was retired, and like many in our area, had become an Uber driver to fill his time. My husband and I describe airplane seats as our second home since we travel frequently to fulfill our purposes. Paul had become our friend. We usually joked about how I am chronically late and overpacked. Once in the car and on our way, I asked, "Paul, are you okay?"

"No," he replied. "I'm worried about my mother. Remember how I moved her here so I could watch over her? It isn't going well." He then proceeded to tell me about his eighty-eight-year-old mother's battle with dementia.

Dementia patients typically experience a gradual decline for several years, followed by a sudden precipitous drop in mental function and physical ability. This abrupt change often leads to panic in those who love them. This was the situation in which Paul found himself.

Having his mom in the house next door had been a great arrangement for a while. He was able to keep a close eye on her and her beloved Chihuahua and offer regular help. But then her dementia began to progress quickly. She lost control of bodily functions and experienced multiple episodes of delirium. She had been hospitalized several times for urinary tract infections (UTIs).

Paul and his wife suddenly found themselves on the caregiving roller coaster. Each day was draining mentally, physically, and emotionally. They remained determined to keep Paul's mom at home because of the promises he had made. With each visit to the ED and each hospital stay, she would show slight, temporary improvement. But she never returned to her previous baseline, which was already poor. Paul was exhausted and unsure of what to do next.

"I know she would hate this for herself and for us," he said, his voice full of emotion. "And I would never want to put my kids through this."

I recognized in Paul the common inner turmoil family members face when they find themselves in this place of helplessness and guilt. The guilt can stem from many things. It can originate in the thought, *I should have prepared better for such a time as this.* Or it can arise from the thought, *My loved one would be better off if he or she could simply pass peacefully and be done with all this suffering.*

If that last sentence hits a little too close to home, know you are not alone. No one wants to see a loved one pass away, but they also do not want to see someone they love struggle and suffer. Paul was in this awful place, and it was breaking his heart. Guilt ate holes in him while love poured out.

He was living in *the waiting place.*

The Mystery of the Waiting Place

Most kinds of waiting are distasteful. End-of-life waiting is unnerving at best, scary at worst. But at least we do not have to wait in vain. We can make the most of this waiting time. It is the time for healthcare providers and family members to show love and care. It is a time for patients to tie up loose ends, mend fences, and say words that need to be said. It can also be a time to worship.

Like Paul, a dear friend of mine from Rwanda was in the waiting place with her mother. She and her ten siblings rotated through sitting with their mother as her bodily functions began to fail. They were unsure what to do during this time. Should they try other doctors, other hospitals, other countries?

After listening for a while, it became clear to me that their beloved mother was dying, and aggressive interventions were not warranted. I suggested they begin a diary of their mother's wisdom and what she would like them to remember. Unlike Paul's mother, whose dementia clouded her memories, my friend's mother and her children used the waiting place to remember triumphs, tragedies, joys, sorrows, strengths, and weaknesses. Each child treasured the blessing she spoke and the faith she imparted to them. She died quietly in the darkness of the night, a good death, a gentle soul returning home.

This family came to appreciate the waiting place. But other families struggle with this delay in departure. Their grief and exhaustion overwhelm them. When I have patients who linger much longer than expected, I ask family members, "Is there anyone else your loved one may need to see or whose presence they may need to feel so that they may rest?" Sometimes, it is the prodigal son or the cousin he or she played with when younger.

While God is preparing the patient's heavenly home, he often desires for the circle of relationship to go unbroken. I don't believe this is just for the benefit of the patient who will soon enter his presence but also for those left behind who may not understand the depth and breadth of God's love for them. He desires to heal their hearts as well.

In my friend Paul's waiting place with his mother, he wasn't just struggling with saying goodbye. He also grappled with which of his mother's treatments should be continued and which should be stopped. Treatment with antibiotics may have resolved his mother's UTIs. But even if successful, winning the small battle against a recurring infection was not going to reverse the outcome in the bigger war against dementia. The circumstances would go from bad to worse.

Some would see withholding antibiotics in such a scenario as hastening the end of life. Others, however, specify in their ACP directives that such treatments be given only when they can extend the patient's life with a quality of life the patient would desire.

Choosing not to do a treatment per the patient's wishes is significantly different than physician-assisted suicide, frequently entitled medical assistance in dying (MAID). MAID is the intentional prescribing of medication that will result in the patient's death. Declining treatment, however, has an unknown outcome; the patient's symptoms and life expectancy are unpredictable. It is still a difficult decision, especially in the absence of an ACP.

As we approached the airport, I said, "Paul, you are a good son. It's time to get hospice involved and let them help you with these hard decisions. Sometimes the best decision is not to keep fighting in vain for life but to focus on dying well. It is that time for your mom." I gave him contact information for two of my favorite local hospice providers and ended our time with a hug.

Paul was a good son, and he anticipated heaven on behalf of his mother. He knew how much he would miss her, but he imagined her without pain and suffering and was thankful for their shared eternity.

The Hard Hard

The second section of the Five Wishes document encourages participants not only to *think about* but to *spell out* the kinds of medical treatment they want and do not want in the event they cannot speak for themselves. I call this the *hard hard.* Nothing about these circumstances is easy.

Even with the most thorough ACP and plan, and even with deep and abiding faith, this section describes events we can't imagine. But for families arriving here without an ACP, it can be disastrous. Please, please, please have a plan. You will not regret it.

Wish 2: My Wish for the Kind of Medical Treatment I Want and Do Not Want

In this part of the Five Wishes document, you are encouraged to write an opening paragraph. On mine, I was detailed. "You should keep in mind as my caregiver that I believe my life is precious and I deserve to be treated with dignity. Therefore, when the time comes that I am too sick to speak for myself, I want the following wishes—and any other directives I have given—to be respected and followed.

"If I am not expected to have a meaningful recovery, I would not wish to be placed on or continue with artificial life support. *Meaningful* to me means the ability to communicate with those I love. I would like my healthcare proxy to seek a second medical opinion. If both primary and secondary opinions agree with the plan I have discussed with my healthcare proxy, then proceed accordingly. My one final request: I don't want to be in pain."

I have a very clear picture of my wishes. It is because of my longtime work in medicine and because I'm in my latter decades. Fortunately, the Five Wishes plan provides guidance for decision-making. These are some highlights and examples of wishes people make in this section:

"I do not want anything done or omitted by my doctors or nurses with the intention of taking my life."

This statement is not in reference to either active or passive euthanasia. Rather, it is meant for a time when you cannot speak for yourself. Not all circumstances result in an obvious answer.

One of the most complex situations regarding a healthcare proxy is in the setting of dementia, as in the story of my friend Paul and his mother. If the patient has dementia and you are a healthcare proxy, it is crucial to determine triggering events when a healthcare proxy should intervene. I describe in Resource A at the back of the book when decisions should be shared.

"I want to be offered food and fluids by mouth and to be kept clean and warm."

The desire to be kept clean and warm at the end of life seems obvious. Who does not want that? The issue of food and fluids *by mouth*, however, can be problematic.

I have seen loved ones desperately attempt to feed or give fluids to an actively dying patient, and that results in aspiration of the fluid into the lungs. Violent coughing ensues and both patient and family member are in distress. A better, alternative approach is mouth care with moistened mouth swabs, which effectively comforts the patient.

As life reaches its end, it is common for the patient to have coarse, wet-sounding breathing. This is often called a death rattle. This is normal. There are medicines to diminish the fluid secretions, but do not ask for suction. It is traumatizing to the patient and ineffective in the end. To help you prepare for the possibilities that can occur at the end of life, I encourage you to read Resource F, which describes the timeline of signs and symptoms that may occur during the last three months of life.

Additionally, families may choose to apply lotion gently to the skin. Compassionate touch is a beautiful gift and a loving way to care for a patient. This is true even for the comatose patient. I have had many spouses join their loved one in the hospital bed, even in the ICU, as they prepare for the long goodbye sigh, the moment of final exhalation.

In my Five Wishes document, I have added, "As long as I have breath, please talk to me, touch me, and play my favorite worship music. I want to praise my way home." We will talk about this in more detail when we get to Wish 4.

"I want to be clear on what *life support* means to me."

I particularly value this statement because "life support" can mean very different things to different people. What's more, with chronic diseases that gradually worsen, the concept of life support can shift and change over time. An example of this is the patient I described in the introduction to this book—the one who so affected me with her wish for a "good death."

Early in her disease process, she made it clear that she did not want life support that included CPR or mechanical ventilation (an artificial breathing machine). However, with the advanced suffering she was experiencing by the time of our conversation, she had modified her wishes to request no life support beyond tending to her basic comforts.

In a perfect world, these changing desires would be discussed with one's primary care clinician well in advance. But the situations leading to such changing desires often occur during a time of hospitalization, and the ensuing discussions generally take place with strangers. We've talked about the benefits of knowledge. Understanding the medical jargon associated with a serious illness will help you navigate decision-making. I have included a dictionary for serious illness terms in Resource G.

If you have questions about these decisions, schedule an appointment with your clinician or his or her designee for further discussion.

Wishes for Extreme Scenarios

The Five Wishes plan presents four circumstances in which your healthcare proxy will need to make decisions on your behalf. It explores these through questions and options. This enables you to spell out your desires in situations where you are:

- Close to death
- Comatose
- Comatose with brain damage
- In a persistent vegetative state

As you consider these agonizing scenarios, remember the "right" answers are *your* answers. Yet this does not change the fact that determining what is right for you is often difficult. This is especially true if you are younger and are completing this document when death seems like a remote concept. But considering the prospect of death brings clarity to life. And don't we all need a little more clarity?

If you are currently in a grave situation (either as a patient or as a healthcare proxy for one who is critically ill), you are likely to interact daily with experienced physicians and nurses who can answer your questions. If they cannot or will not give you the information you need, ask for a second opinion. It is your right. You can also ask for a clinical social worker, a palliative care nurse, or a hospice nurse. We will discuss the difference between palliative care and hospice care in future chapters. For now, here are some options for extreme scenarios.

If I'm Close to Death . . .

While the choice in this scenario might seem obvious, let me give you a real-life example that shows the complexity of this decision.

While mall-walking with his wife, Mr. L collapsed. A security guard began cardiopulmonary resuscitation (CPR) while a bystander called 911. The ambulance and emergency medical technicians arrived promptly and shocked his heart into a normal rhythm. Mrs. L stood by tearfully, trembling in the arms of a stranger.

Resuscitated and on life support, Mr. L was rushed by paramedics to our hospital, where our team of nurses and doctors worked to stabilize him. Meanwhile, Mrs. L waited alone, nervous and fearful.

I stepped out to talk with Mrs. L after a few minutes. When she saw me, she stood up so quickly that her purse tumbled to the floor.

I helped her gather up her spilled items and sat down with her. I informed her that her husband was stable, and we spoke about what had happened at the mall. Her eyes brimming with tears, Mrs. L said, "I am so thankful. May I see him?"

"Of course!" I replied. I led her into the ICU and to her husband's room. She must have been shocked. The love of her life had IVs going into both limbs. He had tubes in his mouth, one delivering breath, the other draining his stomach of bile. The various machines were producing a cacophony of rhythmic sounds, while medical personnel swirled about his bed.

At the center of this hurricane of intense medical activity, Mr. L lay still, his chest barely moving up and down. While a nurse continued working on the other side of the bed, Mrs. L stepped over and gently touched her husband's face. She called his name. No response.

"Can he hear me? Will he be okay?" she asked, her eyes watery and hopeful.

"He was starting to wake up when he arrived, which is a very good sign," I said. "For now, we need to keep him sedated until we're sure he will remain stable. We do believe that patients may hear when they are in this condition, although they don't always remember what they heard. We also need to keep him on the breathing machine while we determine what happened to him."

Without warning, she set down her purse and began to wring her hands and cry. I gave her a hug, figuring her emotions were due to sheer relief after the intense panic of the past few hours. I was wrong.

"He has cancer . . . prostate cancer," she blurted out. "It's bad. It has spread throughout his body. We filled out a form, and he said he does *not* want life support. Is that what this is? I am supposed to be his . . . um, um, person . . . what do you call it? It's like an attorney, but that's not it. Oh, I don't know what I am supposed to do! He said no life support."

Her voice revealed a rising panic as her internal conflict became overwhelming. "But I'm not ready. I didn't say goodbye. We were just walking and then he crumpled to the floor. I didn't say goodbye. I didn't know what to do. I'm not ready to let him go."

"You did exactly what anyone would have done in these circumstances," I reassured her. "I would have done the same thing, even knowing what I know now. I don't believe his prostate cancer is what caused him to collapse. He had an irregular heart rhythm that the EMTs were able to shock back to normal. The best news is that he was already starting to wake up when he got here. My guess is that we'll be able to get him off machines in the next twenty-four hours. We can then ask him if he wants us to further investigate the cause of his heart issue. If so, we'll consult a cardiologist.

"If I'm wrong and he does not wake up soon, we can talk again about removing the machines. Mrs. L, as a healthcare proxy, it's hard to be sure of what to do in emergencies like this. But this is exactly what I would have done if he were my husband. You are doing the best you can."

Her shoulders, which were hunched around her ears, dropped slowly with relief. "Thank you so much," she said. "I needed to hear that. I just want to keep walking with him for as long as I can. Our daughter is on her way. She'll help me."

I hugged her frail, trembling body and was surprised by her strength as she hugged me too. We understood each other at that moment, two women who deeply love their husbands.

I will always remember this case. It was not for how it started, but for how it ended. About a month later, I was at the mall doing some back-to-school shopping, and I almost ran into Mr. and Mrs. L (literally) as I exited a store. We hugged and exchanged greetings, after which they walked quickly away, hands tightly clasped (they were only on lap three of five, and time was a-ticking).

I smiled and thought, *I love my job sometimes.*

In a scenario like this one, it is vital that two healthcare professionals agree that a patient is close to death. Though Mr. L had cancer, it was not the cause of his cardiac arrest. Therefore, by relying on not one but two clinicians (myself and the cardiologist), Mrs. L made the best decision while still honoring her husband's wishes.

If I'm Comatose . . .

This second scenario is more difficult to navigate. The word *coma* can mean different things to different people. It is intuitive to know that it is serious. But people typically think of thrilling stories where a person was comatose but then suddenly awakened and returned to a normal life. Despite these successes, some do not survive a coma.

All comas are not equal. There are many causes for a coma. The prognosis is different depending on patient factors (age, gender, health issues) and the cause of the coma.

This place in an ACP should be read and reread. If you are going through the Five Wishes, pay special attention to the wording (note my emphasis of certain words and phrases): "If my doctor *and* another healthcare professional *both decide* . . . [I am] *not expected to wake up or recover* and I have *brain damage, and life-support treatment would only delay the moment of my death, then . . .*"

A coma often follows a traumatic accident or catastrophic illness. As you decide on this question for yourself in the comfort of your home, and ideally with family members, the answer may seem straightforward. When sitting in an ICU waiting anxiously for the morning doctor to give you an update on your loved one, a clear decision may elude you. If you are the healthcare proxy, you may be asked if you believe the patient would want to continue life support based upon their ACP.

This is why families and healthcare proxies should have multiple copies of a patient's ACP readily available. Most clinical settings will ask if the patient has a completed living will or ACP at the point of entry. This simple act ensures that the clinicians caring for you or your loved one can read specific directives and determine when the criteria of the various wishes have been met. This helps them give wise counsel when it is most needed. Ultimately, the decision is made by the healthcare proxy because he or she represents the voice of the patient.

As previously mentioned, modern medicine's increased use of machines to prolong survival has had a dehumanizing effect. Over time, nurses, doctors, and even family members can begin to see patients impersonally. When artificial life support enters the picture, it is not uncommon to see indelicate life-and-death discussions take place *over the bed of the patient.*

Your loved one may have awareness of the discussion at hand but no ability to speak or react. I have seen doctors and family members confer loudly just outside the room of a dying patient. This should never happen. It is always preferable to request a family consultation room for these conversations. This directive can also be included in an ACP as written text.

Recent studies have revealed that "familiar auditory training techniques" (the recorded voices of family members played regularly) resulted in increased neural activity in language areas of the brain that respond to auditory stimuli.[1] In simpler terms, the areas of the brain that process hearing showed increased activity in the area that interprets language. This study was on patients in a coma due to acute traumatic brain injury. But indicators of auditory processing (hearing) have been found in other types of comas, in advanced dementia patients, and in those who are actively dying up to the point of death. They can still hear you.

If I'm Comatose with Brain Damage . . .

In this circumstance, one is not expected to wake up or recover. Brain damage may occur with trauma but also with a variety of other causes, including lack of oxygen to the brain for extended periods of time.

You may decide in this situation not to be placed on life support. You may also choose to be placed on life support temporarily and then be removed if meaningful recovery is not expected. I previously described that meaningful recovery for me was the ability to communicate. You may choose a different parameter, but include this in your written request.

Regardless, it is difficult for healthcare proxies and family members to make this decision on your behalf in a clinical setting. For family members and proxies, if a patient makes that choice in his or her ACP, *all* family members should honor and support it. Patients with a severe or terminal illness may feel they have lost their autonomy as their illness progresses. Giving them the freedom to express opinions and choices is crucial. Lamenting with them as they make the decision yet supporting them is the greatest expression of love.

Even when loved ones have prepared for the possibility of such a terrible moment, both in writing and in verbal consultations with doctors, there is no way to prepare for the avalanche of emotions that accompanies such emergencies. Every circumstance is different, each person is unique, and each relationship is one of a kind. You may wish to specify that if doctors agree that your prognosis is not hopeful, family members should be given adequate time to say their goodbyes.

Also consider the question, "Can others be saved through my death?" Having had the grateful recipients of donated organs as patients, I have witnessed the hope organ donation delivers.

I have cared for families navigating the decision to donate organs from their loved one who is brain dead. It is never easy, yet I have seen faith in Christ become the sinew that holds families together. Decision-making with prayer and the Holy Spirit brings comfort and discernment. It is in these times that anticipating heaven is hope realized and faith actualized. God's Word remains true no matter the decisions made:

> God will redeem my soul from the power of the
> grave,
> For He shall receive me. (Psalm 49:15)

If I'm in a Persistent Vegetative State . . .

Here we're talking about situations of irreversible, permanent, and severe brain damage. The condition known as *persistent vegetative state* can only be diagnosed after four weeks.[2] At that time, a diagnosis of "not expected to recover" depends on the cause of the condition.

Be cautious as you hear this term, and please do not use the phrase "he or she will be a vegetable." If you cannot remember the medical phrase "persistent vegetative state," simply say, "not expected to wake up." In Resource D, I discuss in more detail *persistent vegetative state*. In this section of the Five Wishes document, you may add additional directives under the heading *Another Condition Under Which I Do Not Wish to Be Kept Alive.* Let me illustrate with a patient story.

"Goodbye, My Love"

Mr. G was frequently admitted to the hospital due to severe lung disease. He required a ventilator on most admissions. This treatment purchased him a little more time and enabled him to return home. Though he fought hard, his lungs and body weakened.

It became more difficult to wean him from the ventilator with each admission. Each admission grew longer, each stay at home, shorter. Mr. G ultimately made the decision that he did not want the ventilator anymore. He chose for himself the designation Do Not Resuscitate, or DNR.

Mr. G's change in wishes was communicated to his healthcare providers. One winter afternoon I was called to the ED to admit him after he presented in respiratory distress. He remained firm in his decision not to be intubated and placed on the ventilator. He did agree to try a BiPAP—a respiratory assist device that delivers breath through a tight-fitting mask. It is one step away from a ventilator, but not considered life support.

We rolled Mr. G into the elevator and crowded in on either side of his stretcher. The respiratory therapist delivered breaths by squeezing a soft rubber bag that filled the mask with air. I stood on the other side holding both his hands with mine. They were cold. Mrs. G stood next to me and tried to soothe him as she rubbed his legs.

We arrived at the ICU and Mrs. G went directly to the waiting room. She knew this room all too well.

"I will bring you in as soon as we get him settled," I said to her as the double doors of the ICU swung open.

After transferring him to the bed, we exchanged the bag for the ventilator, still delivering oxygenated air through the mask. He immediately began to pull on the mask and the straps that held it in place.

"Mr. G, you must leave the mask in place. Your oxygen levels drop when you move it."

His eyes were wide, panicked. He had not looked this uncomfortable even when awake and on the ventilator.

"Are you sure you don't want us to put you on the ventilator?" I asked, fully expecting him to say yes.

"No, no! Claus . . . Claus . . . tro . . . pho . . . bic!" He gasped with each syllable. "My . . . wife . . ." His voice trailed off, and I understood what he wanted and needed. I told the nurse to get her as I held both of his hands once again.

"Please, please keep the mask on, and we will get you something to help you relax." His eyes softened as his wife arrived and rushed up to the other side of the bed. She took one hand.

"I'm . . . read . . . y," he finally announced to his wife. "I know . . . where I'm goin' and rea . . . ready . . . to get there." The last sentence was expelled with every effort given.

He had lived anticipating heaven for some time. He had no fear, just confidence.

With tears sliding down her cheeks, she gave a nod that was nearly imperceptible. She was ready to let him go. His oxygen was switched to a nasal cannula. He was made comfortable and given morphine to diminish his "air hunger."

His wife held his hand that afternoon until a nurse called me back to the room. We watched his heart rate slow and finally stop.

As Mrs. G gave Mr. G one last kiss, her tears were gone. His long struggle and suffering were over, and it was time for rest, for both husband and wife.

Mr. G's death was one of the bravest I have witnessed. I pray that my death will be so courageous. I pray that I will have a song in my heart and God's name on my lips. I also pray for every person who reads these words who is facing the end, that you can step confidently into eternity praising your way home.

We have covered difficult topics in this chapter, many of which may never come to pass in your or your family's lifetime. My friend and driver, Paul, said goodbye to his mother, a family in Rwanda made use of the waiting place, and Mr. G slipped confidently into eternity. As you, your family, and your loved ones wrestle through these decisions, know that being prepared avoids infinitely more anguish.

> *We are confident, yes, well pleased rather to be absent from the body and to be present with the Lord.*
>
> 2 CORINTHIANS 5:8

seven

CARE AND CARING

Death is no more than passing from one room into another.
But there's a difference for me, you know.
Because in that other room I shall be able to see.
HELEN KELLER

Ron was a giant of a man, both in stature and personality. He laughed with his whole body, like a rumbling volcano just before it erupted. It was contagious. He was known throughout our community for his fun-loving sense of humor and his generosity of spirit. All these years later, I don't know whether to laugh or to cry when I think of him and some of his antics.

Ron had lost weight and had a gnawing pain in his abdomen. He felt pretty sure the aspirin powders he had been taking for headaches had caused an ulcer. He decided to tell Mary, his wife, about it one day.

His wife chided him, "I told you that you had been taking too many."

He chuckled, "You know I am twice your size, Mary—of course,

I'm gonna take twice as many. Plus, Mary, my noggin is four times yours, so I have big headaches." He nearly doubled over, laughing at his own cleverness, as she wrote herself a reminder to schedule a doctor's appointment the next day.

Cancer hit him hard and fast. It was a sucker punch to the belly—quite literally the pancreas.

In a matter of months, Ron appeared to have lost half his body weight. His sallow skin hung loosely on top of atrophied muscle. His sense of humor remained, although the energy for a good old belly laugh had dissipated along with the other half of his body.

Ron rapidly comprehended the writing on the wall, while Mary obsessed over alternative therapies, treatments, and clinical trials. He began to anticipate heaven, while Mary spent hours and hours praying for a healing. Prayer chains were started from church to church and city to city.

The cancer spread at alarming speed, and the pain began to rob him of . . . him. Pain pills and pain patches took the sharp edges from this thief named cancer, but the dull presence of pain during the day was unleashed at night, and sleep eluded him.

Ron's faith stood strong despite the physical suffering he endured. He began to read Scripture more and pray more, and for the first time, he worshiped from the depth of his soul. While his physical body diminished, his spiritual body grew in stature. He lived looking to eternity and a new body that would not betray him.

Meanwhile, Mary's grief became as destructive as Ron's cancer. She could not understand how her loving God, to whom she had been devoted her entire life, had now seemingly failed her. Her faith was faltering, and she began to shake her fist at God figuratively. She stopped asking others for prayer. She knew she loved God, yet she was angry at his silence.

The truth is, God was speaking to Mary, but she didn't want to hear what he had to say. Meanwhile, Ron heard every word he spoke.

"God, I'm Angry!"

Mary's and Ron's story is not unusual amid the grieving of dying. Their faith was deeply affected by the crisis of cancer. Yet they were affected differently. It may be easy to talk about faith, but its strength is fully known when it is tested. I have seen many discover inner strength and peace amid their crises. It was what they needed at the exact moment they needed it. Faith in the trenches is a beautiful gift from God.

For others, faith provides a place to focus their pain, questions, confusion, and even anger. We cannot be angry at God and not believe in him. Our Father God can receive each of our emotions as we cry out for answers. He understands our pain. He grieves with the brokenhearted and the afflicted.

> He has not despised nor abhorred the affliction of the
> afflicted;
> Nor has He hidden his face from Him;
> But when He cried to Him, He heard. (Psalm 22:24)

He hears you.

> I will be glad and rejoice in Your mercy,
> For You have considered my trouble;
> You have known my soul in adversities. (Psalm 31:7)

He knows you.

> The Lord is near to those who have a broken heart,
> And saves such as have a contrite spirit. (Psalm 34:18)

He saves you.

"I Wish, I Wish, I Wish"

The last three of the Five Wishes are practical steps we can take to ensure the waiting time is not spent in vain, whether you are waiting in faith or feel your faith being tested. It is a way to focus in the face of pain. These wishes cover the important issues of comfort, dignity, and legacy.

Wish 3: My Wish for How Comfortable I Want to Be

For some, the dying process includes pain. But the dying process can also include respiratory distress, nausea, excessive oral secretions, or anxiety. In the final stage of life, alleviating pain and suffering adequately and compassionately is the most important role of the clinician.

Many choose to include as part of their ACP an overt statement to the effect of, "I do not want to be in pain. I want my doctor to give me enough medicine to relieve my suffering, even if that means I will be drowsier or sleep more than I would otherwise."

Managing pain and other symptoms for the dying patient can be achieved either in a clinical environment or at home via hospice supervision. The latter arrangement allows patients to spend their final days in familiar surroundings. It also enables families to participate in the loving care of a patient who is dying. Ron and Mary chose to stay at home during his dying journey. Years after Ron's death, Mary was still thankful for their decision to remain in their home when Ron needed it most.

Wish 4: My Wish for How I Want People to Treat Me

I encourage those who are either facing or anticipating death to state overtly in their advance directives the desire to be treated with dignity. Here is why.

Disease is a stalker and a cruel companion. It is also a thief. It robs its victims of autonomy, opportunity, vitality, and longevity. Given enough time, disease even has an insidious way of stealing a person's identity. Those suffering from chronic, long-term illnesses sometimes lose the ability to see themselves as *people*, or even as *patients*. Instead, their whole existence seems defined by their disease.

Ron's sense of humor was legendary and became a source of comfort after his diagnosis. When people in his life felt unsure of what to say or do, he broke the ice with cancer jokes. This helped him cope and not be defined by the life he had but by the life he was making (however short it may have been).

Sometimes this humor in the face of death exasperated Mary. She was mourning his loss before his departure. Loved ones need to be especially sensitive to the needs of both the patient and the primary caregiver. Friends spending time with Mary gave her space to express her fears and grief. It takes a village.

This is why dignity for those at the end of life is so important. It is crucial for healthcare providers, caregivers, family members, friends—really, all of society—to see past the ravages of disease to the unique person inside each ailing, failing body and the unique stressors affecting the immediate family. While we want to treat sick bodies with the best medicines and therapies, it is vital that we also treat suffering souls with the utmost respect and dignity.

Those at the end of life can be as helpless as a child entering the world, and therefore they should be treated with extreme gentleness. They are not, however, infants in shriveled bodysuits. They need people to address their physical, mental, emotional, and spiritual needs too.

When I care for dying patients and advise their families, I remember that I will be in that bed one day. I seek to comfort others the way I will one day want to be comforted. As a family member or loved one of a dying patient, it is crucial to have this perspective.

"I want a listening ear."

It is important to remember that each person has lived a life full of moments: breathtaking moments of beauty and joy, life-altering moments of insight, and heartbreaking moments of loss. Showing dignity to the dying means sitting with them, listening to their recollections, and learning from their moments. This is true love, true caring, and true learning.

From experience, I have come to realize a great truth: the dying patient has wisdom that transcends our common daily experience. We must have ears to hear it and hearts willing to accept it. Active listening is a gift to both the dying patient and to us. It honors each person's one-of-a-kind life.

If you are nearing the end of life, I appeal to you: *Please* share your moments. Pass on to us the things you have learned. Do not deprive us of your unique perspective and experience. We need your insight. We need your wisdom to whisper to us in those hard but holy moments. We know you are anticipating heaven, but while you are here, share with us what was meaningful in your life, as well as your regrets. You and your life experience have profound benefits for those you leave behind.

As friends and family visited Ron, he shared stories from his life, prompting raucous laughter and sacred moments. Sometimes Mary would join these trips down memory lane. Other times she'd step out of the house and get her hair done or go grocery shopping, appreciating slivers of time with normalcy.

Another patient called this sweet time "the long goodbye." It is an opportunity to record the meaningful memories, lessons learned, challenges faced, and victories celebrated. Audio, video, or written recordings extend the essence of a life for future generations.

Mary did this for Ron by keeping a book of photos captioned with Ron's words or those said about him. It was shared at his funeral, and she still treasures this book of memories.

"I want to die in my home, if that is possible."

We have become a society where dying and death have been relegated largely to clinical settings such as ICUs or skilled nursing wings at hospitals and nursing homes. Sometimes, because of medical circumstances, this is unavoidable. Often, however, in the case of terminal diseases, spending one's final days at home is a viable option.

For loved ones, I know bringing your loved one home to die may be the most difficult gift that you will ever give. Even so, it is a gift of immense dignity, beauty, and love. In the next chapter, I will give some guidelines to assist those making these decisions.

Wish 5: My Wish for What I Want My Loved Ones to Know

This last wish of the Five Wishes is really about legacy. What do you want to leave behind? What unexpressed truths do you need to spell out? There is truth in the saying, "Last words are lasting words." This is your opportunity to say those things you most need to say and your loved ones most need to hear.

I know one man who, prior to a trip overseas to a war-torn area, wrote "just in case" letters to his wife and two sons. The experience was powerful and deeply moving. He tried to put into words his deep love for his family and his highest, best hopes for each family member.

Seize the opportunity (while you have it) to pour out your heart on paper. Even as I reread and ponder the import of my own words in my fifth wish, each statement moves me again. I know my answers for this wish may change between today and some future day (if it is my destiny to have a future day). Therefore, whatever you write in this directive should be reexamined often and updated as needed.

My Wish

In my fifth and final wish, I encouraged my family to embrace the following values, actions, reminders, and habits:

- Choose love
- Fear forward
- Forgive
- Live in peace
- Find your purpose
- Laugh daily
- Suffering exists; dwell on joy
- Teach the truth about Jesus Christ
- Celebrate moments

- Respect others
- Grow daily
- Live a meaningful life
- Love God and others deeply
- Have fun

These are the principles I hope to instill in my loved ones and leave behind when I go. What do you hope to leave behind? I encourage you to contemplate what you would like for those you love to remember. Record your thoughts in writing or through a video diary and your perfectly imperfect, big, beautiful life will impact those who follow you.

Whatever you choose, I hope you'll take the time to prepare your plan—with a document like the Five Wishes or another ACP. The Five Wishes concludes with instructions on what to do once you have completed the document. My encouragement is to start early, ask questions, reevaluate as needed, and share your directives with all who need to know.

Your Directive Documents

Whether you opt for the Five Wishes document or another ACP, the intrinsic value of such directives is only seen when they are communicated across all levels and locations of your medical care. Therefore, it is up to you to make sure your combined directive document(s) can be easily accessed by those who are affected by your wishes.

- Keep the original in a safe place in your home and give a copy to family members and your healthcare proxy.

- Give a copy to all your physicians.
- Make a list of those who have the document and who can speak to its validity (if your healthcare proxy is not immediately available).
- If possible, carry a wallet-sized card that indicates that you have an ACP and gives the name and phone number of your healthcare proxy and the location of the original document.
- Keep a copy (hard copy or digital copy) of the document with you when traveling.
- If you are utilizing the Five Wishes, refer to their website periodically for additional resources.
- Update your document. The Five Wishes website has a digital version of the document that can be changed over time and accessed at any time with your name and password. (Giving this information to all the key people in your life is critical in the event of an emergency when it needs to be accessed.)

Your actions now can help others in your family avoid having to grope blindly and helplessly for direction in your final days.

"Jesus, Jesus!"

Mary prayed with her entire being that Ron would be healed. Her initial response was anger for unanswered prayer. But in time and with leaning into Ron's faith and hope of anticipating heaven, she finally accepted God's will. Her faith became her rock once more, and she also began to anticipate heaven, where she would one day reunite with the one she loved and was losing.

In the final week of his life, Ron's pain worsened. As his

healthcare proxy, Mary agreed that controlling his pain was more important than his being awake all the time. She tended to him as she had tended their children when they were babies. She rubbed lotion into his bony limbs. She moistened his dry, cracked tongue with a mouth swab and his lips with Vaseline. She could not help but kiss him with gentle kisses. She sang to him and read the Psalms. Their children came in to join her in his death vigil. While he had had a lot of visitors in the previous six months, the family requested only their pastor and his wife as time grew short.

He woke up less frequently, and as the final time drew near, he did not wake at all. His pain was visible through grimaces and moans, and morphine doses were increased until he would rest. The family gathered around the bed as Mary sat holding his hand.

He startled the entire room when he suddenly sat up in bed with a strength that defied his physical condition. He clapped loudly, looked heavenward, and shouted—*shouted*—"Jesus! Jesus!" Falling back in bed, he shuddered and expelled his final breath.

Mary said much later, "The room was quiet, stunned, and then they all broke out in tears."

It was a big ending for a giant of a man. He is missed deeply, but his imprint on this life remains. His anticipating heaven became a great blessing for his entire family. Nothing prepared them for his exit, yet each was comforted by it.

Your ending moment is known only by God but *living with the end in mind* prepares you and those you love for when that moment occurs. Completing the ACP will help alleviate some of your fears. The next chapters are to help with other fears you may be experiencing by giving you knowledge about the patient's healthcare journey, understanding the power of prayer, miracles, and how to have God as your strength and your portion forever.

If you are a loved one, caregiver, or healthcare proxy, you will also discover more to help you cope and give you hope as God will bring you strength when you need it most.

> *My flesh and my heart fail;*
> *But God is the strength of my heart and my portion forever.*
> PSALM 73:26

Part Two

PREPARING YOUR MIND, HEART, AND SOUL

eight

PARADIGM SHIFTS: ANTICIPATING HEAVEN IN THE STORM

Some of God's greatest mercies are in his refusals. He says no in order that he may, in some way we cannot imagine, say yes.
ELISABETH ELLIOT

Our hospital admits as many tourists as locals because we are situated in a resort community. Some tourists are in the middle of treatments for severe diseases. I am sure that their thinking is along the lines of, *I don't care if I* do *have cancer—I'm going to live my life! I'm taking that long-planned vacation!*

Often these restless souls do not bother telling their oncologists they are slipping down south for a few days of R and R following a chemotherapy treatment. (I cannot blame them. In their shoes, I would do the same.) I am sure they are concerned that their doctors would discourage traveling.

Mrs. R was one such sojourner. She'd been coming to our beaches her entire life. She experienced these beach vacations as a child, with her children, and with her husband once they became empty nesters. This visit, however, was different. In recent months, her "health passport" for the foreign lands of clinical care had been stamped multiple times. Hospitals, treatment centers, and doctor's offices had become a second home back in Indiana. The couple realized this beach trip would be her last.

Sadly, upon arrival in our community, she developed a high fever and needed to be admitted to the hospital. I was her admitting doctor.

When I greeted her, I could sense the strength of her will. She spoke of the blur of all those family vacations. She desired a clearer picture.

She earnestly said, "I have so many memories of my children playing in the sand, the morning sun warming our faces. I didn't come simply to see the ocean. I came to relive those memories in their fullness. I came to sink my toes in the sand, the same sand where my children left so many footprints through the years. I know you must understand."

Immediately, I remembered my own kids running and laughing as the low-tide waves chased them in a game of tag. I thought of the beautiful sunrises that greet me daily, leaving gorgeous reflections—like painted canvases—in tide pools. In my mind's eye, I could see the brilliance of a harvest moon set against the darkness of the sea.

I *did* understand.

Mrs. R spoke of this beauty before saying a single word about how she felt, before we discussed her health. I listened closely because *what people talk about most passionately reveals what they value most deeply.* She was making her priorities known. Cancer had robbed her of many things. It was not going to rob her of this final memory at the beach.

Eventually, we discussed her medical issues. She told me none of the treatments the doctors had tried had worked. She was not expecting a cure or even a slowing of the disease. She knew she didn't have many weeks to survive.

She spoke about her life, her family, her disease, and her decline. Her cancer and her dying helped her articulate her life. She described the chapters that mattered. This trip was meant to close the last chapter; the epilogue would occur at home.

She was quite familiar with her healthcare system at home. But our hospital was a kind of foreign land to her, and I, of course, was a stranger. Her anxious husband stood by as she walked me through her health history.

She expressed confidence that she would return home to her loving family and die with her dreams fulfilled. I marveled at this strong woman. She was yet another patient who would be my teacher. She knew her true condition, but more than knowledge, she had wisdom. She displayed more courage than fear, more peace than worry, more hope than despair. I was immensely inspired by her faith.

My role as her temporary physician changed at that point. I was *not* to keep her in the hospital for some recommended length of time. Nor was I to run multiple tests that would only delay her release. My job was to get her well enough that she might fulfill her dream of enjoying a few last days at the beach before returning home to die.

Unselfish Love

This is what I call a *paradigm shift*. It is a necessary, important change in perspective for physicians and patients. As healthcare providers, we are trained to do everything in our power to battle disease and restore health (or at least maintain health). With our white coats and stethoscopes as our armor, and with new pharmaceuticals and cutting-edge treatments as our weapons, we are always ready to go to war. But sometimes we fight so hard that we lose sight of what we are fighting. If we are not careful, our mission can become data driven, and time can become our number one assessment tool. We can forget that winning the battle doesn't always mean more days but rather better days.

Like all people, Mrs. R had faced multiple paradigm shifts along her health journey. I was witnessing her final shift. She no longer sought treatment that would extend her life. She simply wanted to live her life while she still had it. She wanted to *live while dying.*

Time on the beach was more precious and meaningful to her than getting back a few labs marked WNL (within normal limits). She wanted to experience her heaven on earth while anticipating the heavenly kingdom of God.

The Bible says, "The kingdom of heaven is like treasure hidden in a field, which a man found and hid; and for joy over it he goes and sells all that he has and buys that field" (Matthew 13:44). Mrs. R found her treasure in the memories she relived on the beach.

Conversations about such a paradigm shift require time, active listening, and, most importantly, empathy. In this instance, Mr. R gave his wife all these gifts. Despite lamenting her imminent departure, he chose to love her unselfishly by embracing her dream of what would make for a good death.

His example reminds us that it is vital for family members to recognize when such a paradigm shift is occurring and to support their loved ones through the process. It is equally important for clinicians to note such paradigm shifts and to cooperate.

Since you will likely never hear a physician say, "It's time to make a paradigm shift," let me share some examples of when these changes typically occur. This will also help you develop critical thinking skills when you and your loved ones make choices.

Paradigm Shift 1: From Acute to Chronic

We have all had the experience of a temporary illness. You are healthy one day, but the next morning you wake up with some kind of cold or mild illness. You take some medicine, get some rest, and twenty-four or forty-eight hours later, you are back to normal. In a week, this episode is all but forgotten. It is a health hiccup, a short-term setback.

But perhaps you have reached the age where the people in your life share on a regular basis about different kinds of maladies that are striking them. On social media, you read about another former classmate dying suddenly from a heart attack. You discover that a friend or a neighbor is going in for a follow-up appointment after a suspicious mammogram.

Then you realize it has been two-plus years since you have seen your doctor. You make an appointment and show up for a wellness exam, and you are surprised. Your blood pressure and your cholesterol are higher than they should be. After your "wellness" visit, you do not feel so well anymore.

As a result, you change your diet, start exercising, lose a

few pounds, and once more feel in control of your destiny. You return for your follow-up appointment confident that all shall be well once again. But despite your healthy changes and vigorous efforts, your blood pressure remains high. The doctor counsels you and then calls in a prescription for you to pick up on your way home.

A paradigm shift is occurring. You have enjoyed good health for most of your life. It has been one of the few areas in which you always felt in control. Suddenly, you realize you are not. Despite your disciplined attempts to regain your health, you are now a patient. From now on, you will be one of those poor souls who must take medicine daily. You begin to feel old.

For some, this paradigm shift is traumatic, especially if they have lived under the delusion of being in complete control of their health. Some fight feverishly to regain control and obsessively check their blood pressure at every opportunity. They mistakenly believe that if they can just get the numbers to dip below a certain level, they can stop the medication.

Others feel guilty when they remember the friends with failing health they have not contacted. They then worry, *Is everyone going to forget me in my illness the way I've forgotten others?* Still others take these changes in stride and decide to see the journey forward as getting more interesting.

This last group is the one we should strive to join. Most paradigm shifts of health are less traumatic with practice. If we practice activities that keep us healthy, we will have less guilt. If we practice accepting what we cannot change, we will have more peace. And if we practice gratitude for what we can do, rather than lament what we can't, we will have more joy.

FINDING A GOOD DOCTOR

When Mrs. R entered our hospital, I was a stranger. If you are a patient and you've begun your journey with a stranger for a doctor as well, you may begin to wonder, *Am I with the right doctor?*

It's important to develop good relationships with trustworthy clinicians. But first you must choose. Finding the right doctor may take some time and homework. Begin with finding answers to the two most important questions:

1. **Is a prospective doctor competent?** All physicians, upon completion of training, take the Hippocratic oath,[1] which includes the concept of "doing no harm." How do you determine competency? Examples would be:
   - *Is he or she board-certified?* Visit the website www.certificationmatters.org. Certified doctors have rigorous requirements of continuing education in their specialty to maintain certification.
   - *Is a prospective doctor in good standing with his or her medical board?* The information is readily available through each state's licensing board. Enter your state and board of medicine in your search bar and when you identify the website, there will be a feature to look up doctors by name.
   - *What do other patients say about him or her?* Take the time to look at websites that allow patients to post reviews. As you do, however, realize that a few

unhappy patients do not automatically mean that a doctor is of poor quality. Multiple poor reviews, however, are a warning sign.

- *Does a trusted friend or neighbor regard this doctor as competent?* One of the best approaches to finding a competent doctor is to ask other professionals who they see as a clinician. This is especially helpful if they are directly or indirectly associated with healthcare in your area. Doctors, nurses, dentists, attorneys, and others often have an insight that your neighbor may not have.

  For example, the dental assistant I visit has plenty of wisdom about healthcare in our area, including who to see and who not to see. She sits with patients all day long as she waits for the dentist to return to the room and gets the scoop when someone has had a good or bad healthcare visit.

2. **Is a prospective doctor trustworthy?** Above all, you must have confidence in your physician. You must believe that he or she will always act in your best interests. Trust is either borrowed or earned. Borrowed trust is based on the testimony of someone who has had a personal experience with a doctor and trusts him or her. Earned trust takes time but is ultimately more valuable. It is achieved through positive experience on a repetitive basis. It is not abstract, and it is deeply personal and visceral.

You need to trust that your physician knows when to refer. You need to trust that he or she will send you to doctors they believe in. You need to trust that your clinician will not simply tell you what you want to hear or give you what you want to receive. Most of all, you need to trust that your clinician cares.

When your trusted doctor proposes a procedure, plan of care, or treatment, he or she won't mind when you ask questions about its necessity, safety, alternatives, and cost. If trust is present, you will have a more satisfactory doctor-patient relationship.

If you cannot readily find a good doctor, consider the following options:

- If the doctor you wanted has a full patient roster, ask if they have a physician extender who is taking patients. These are either *physician assistants* or *nurse practitioners.* They are present in most practices and are under direct physician supervision. You can also ask if the physician has a waiting list for new patients.
- Some practices are affiliated with training programs. Recent graduates from residency and fellowship programs often stay in the area in which they trained and are eager to fill their appointment times.
- Consider a health maintenance organization (HMO) as your insurance and care providers. The gatekeepers of an HMO are primary care physicians who delegate to specialists as needed. Make sure you understand their process and costs for in-network and out-of-network care.
- Visit your local hospital websites, which should have a feature for finding affiliated doctors.

- Ask your insurance company or Medicare for recommendations. You can also visit the following websites to identify physicians in your area:
    - www.medicare.gov
    - www.ama-assn.org
    - www.certificationmatters.org

  These options can give you a good start.

Paradigm Shift 2: From Chronic to Disability

The shift from a chronic disease to disability is a dramatic one when the emotional consequences are measured. It is one I encounter often in my patients. It's also one of the hardest to accept. A *chronic* medical condition is generally defined as "lasting longer than one year and requiring ongoing medical attention or limits activities of daily living or both."[2] A *disability* is described by the World Health Organization as:

- "Impairment in a person's body structure or function, or mental function."
- "Activity limitation, such as difficulty seeing, hearing, walking, or problem solving."
- "Participation restriction in normal daily activities."[3]

Not all chronic illnesses lead to disability, and not all disabilities are the result of a chronic illness. But some cases of chronic illness that lead to disability carry an additional weight of deep regret. The story of one of my patients comes to mind.

Mr. C was a thin, scraggly patient struggling to complete full sentences when I first met him. Every third or fourth breath, he inhaled deeply to catch his breath. He picked at his fingertips, which were discolored by years of tobacco use. He looked sickly—miserable. My heart went out to him immediately.

"I can tell it's hard for you to breathe when you talk," I said. "Would it be okay if I asked your wife some questions about your health?" He nodded with relief, laid his head back, and closed his eyes.

I learned that from a young age, Mr. C had worked hard, sometimes two jobs, so that his wife could stay home with their three daughters. Like most of his coworkers, he smoked on a regular basis. He only started cutting back on smoking at the age of sixty, when he began to experience mild shortness of breath with activity and when he began having recurring bronchitis. His wife and daughters constantly pleaded with him to quit, to no avail.

"How much do you smoke?" I asked. He sat up slightly, sheepishly looked at his wife, and gasped, "Half pack. Don't inhale."

"Okay, we can talk more about that later," I said, moving on to my other questions.

After my assessment, I looked at Mr. C and then at the women in his life who stood anxiously by his bedside. "Your symptoms are consistent with infection. There is evidence of pneumonia developing in your right lung. Because your oxygen level is low, we need to admit you to the hospital to give you IV antibiotics, breathing treatments, and oxygen. You will likely need to be in the hospital for a minimum of two days; however, it is possible that we may need to keep you longer. We just want to make sure you are safe before we send you home."

At this, one of his daughters stepped forward and announced, "The urgent care doctor told him that he most likely has emphysema or C-O-P-D." (She placed great emphasis on each letter of the acronym that's shorthand for chronic obstructive pulmonary disease.)

"He was supposed to get further testing," she continued, "but he won't listen to us, or even to the urgent care doctor. And he *refuses* to find a primary care doctor for a diagnosis!" Her voice was getting higher and louder. "Will you please tell him he has to find a doctor and *quit smoking*? Mom is worried all the time. He won't listen, and I don't live close enough to make him do the right thing!"

All the women in the room stood a little taller when she finished. In fact, they looked like human exclamation points.

Mr. C stared weakly at these formidable female forces in his life, each wearing an expression somewhere between hostility and loving concern. I thought, *I bet he wishes he had a cigarette right about now.* My instincts were right; a couple of days later, he was caught smoking in the stairwell. At discharge, I referred Mr. C to a local primary care physician whom I trusted, a really "good doctor."

He did not go.

And his condition went from chronic to disability.

Do you relate to some aspect of this story? Do you feel guilt or shame that a habit you acquired ultimately resulted in the disease *you were warned about*? Do you want to ignore the problem (and the concerned loved ones) until it reaches a crisis point?

Perhaps you relate to the women in this story. They clearly love their husband and father but are frustrated with his seeming lack of care for himself. Is your loved one not seeking medical attention when he or she has been told? This is an extremely common occurrence.

What should you do?

What if Mr. C had not smoked and had a severe lung illness from some other condition? He would not feel guilt or shame and therefore avoid doctors and hospitals like the plague. The wife and daughters would be more comforting. The stairwell would not be filled with smoke, and everyone would be more comfortable developing a plan upon departure from the hospital.

As difficult as this may be to hear, patients and families must start from the diagnosis, not what caused it. It ultimately leads to better emotional health for all concerned. But this was not the case with Mr. C as he transitioned from chronic disease to disability.

The next time I saw Mr. C, the family had good news and bad news. The good news was that Mr. C had finally quit smoking. The bad news was that his decision came far too late; his lungs were permanently damaged. Due to his advancing COPD, the formerly active Mr. C was required to always wear oxygen.

This embarrassed him. He rarely left his house except for hospital stays every three or four months. After each episode, his functional status declined.

Through the years and hospital stays, Mr. C and I had many talks. This was *not* the retirement for which they had saved and planned. He battled depression. The things he had previously enjoyed served only to remind him of the abilities he had once had but now had lost.

His friendships withered as he began to reject calls for visits. "I don't want to slow them down," he always explained. In time, the days and nights blurred together, sleep being his only escape from his sad thoughts. Mrs. C and their daughters watched helplessly. They weren't sure what to do. Their beloved husband and father was withering away in front of their eyes.

What should they do? What should you do if you are also living with a chronic or disabling disease?

FACING A DISABILITY

- **Rely on your doctor.** Use the principles below to confirm you have the right doctor(s). Your primary care physician is the "quarterback" of your team. Should a specialist be needed, this primary care physician will refer you to someone well qualified to diagnose and treat your specific condition. If possible, use a pediatrician, family practitioner, internist, or geriatrician. A geriatrician is a doctor for the aging population. They are particularly helpful if you:
  - Are experiencing functional decline or disability
  - Have multiple medical conditions or multiple medications
  - Have diseases associated with aging such as dementia, osteoporosis, or incontinence
- **Educate yourself.** Visit the Patient Advocate Foundation at www.patientadvocate.org for educational resources.
- **Address your symptoms.** You and your family should consider whether you are a candidate for palliative care. *Palliative care* focuses on management of symptoms for care, but not cure. This can be your only medical care or can be in addition to traditional treatments focused on cure. As with hospice care discussed below, the website www.nhpco.org has resources regarding palliative care. Ask your clinician if you would qualify.

- **Make choices.** You can maintain a sense of autonomy even if you only make small choices in your day. This can include meal choices, free-time choices, connecting with old and new friends, time with God, and time alone. Your state of mind is the ultimate choice of autonomy. Gratefulness, joy, and love are willful expressions of God within you made available through the practice of engaging the Holy Spirit. This gift cannot be taken from you, but you must choose it daily, sometimes hourly.
- **Monitor emotional health closely.** Physical disease often results in changes in emotional health. If you are the patient, undoubtedly you experience a multitude of emotions with each doctor visit or hospital stay. Talking with those you love, a pastor, friend, or your clinician is important for receiving the care that is available.

  The patient's loved ones should be mindful of the patient's emotions and engage dialogue about how they are feeling. Patients sometimes don't want to add their emotional burden to their beloved families and may not bring it up on their own.

  If a loved one facing a disability doesn't want to talk and you still have concerns, it would be appropriate to speak to clinicians about your concerns. But in most countries, you would need to have permission from the patient due to privacy laws. Families, friends, and caregivers must also consider their own emotional health and seek help if necessary.

  Some changes to look out for include:

  - Prolonged sadness, irritability, and anxiousness

- Feelings of isolation even when surrounded by loved ones
- The inability to enjoy activities previously enjoyed (especially when physical symptoms are not the limiting factor)
- Sleeping or eating excessively or not enough
- Thoughts of death or suicide (or suicide attempts)
- Unusual pain that is not related to the primary illness

The link between chronic illness and depression is more complex than merely feeling sad about a diagnosis. It includes a biological relationship.[4] Untreated depression, for example, can result in increased risk of cardiovascular disease, diabetes, stroke, and dementia, to name but a few.[5] Given Mr. C's severe mood swings and behavioral changes as his disease progressed, care for his mental health was as important as care for his physical health.

- **Examine your fears.** In our humanity, we share common fears when we approach the prospect of our own mortality. Many of the fears you may experience are normal. Some can be resolved by having knowledge of what to expect. Others have less power over you when you talk about them. Christians are not immune to fear. But it is the dying process we fear most rather than death. We can see death as necessary to experience the heaven we have anticipated. Examining your own fears is courageous, and sharing them authentically is freeing.
- **Avoid isolation at all costs.** Isolation not only exacerbates depression and anxiety, but it also may result in

physical conditions such as high blood pressure, dementia, heart disease, and weakened immune function.[6]

- **Use all services available.** Access all ancillary services for healthcare. Examples would be cardiac rehabilitation, physical therapy, and pulmonary rehabilitation. Discuss with your clinician if you are a candidate for one of these services to obtain a referral.
- **Know you are not alone.** Despite all the people surrounding you, you may still feel alone. If you are feeling crushed, cry out to God. At times I have felt so brokenhearted, I didn't even know how to pray. I would wake during the middle of the night and lay my head on my Bible. God met me there. He will meet you too.

Some of the patients I have treated in the paradigm shift from chronic to disability have become mentors and even heroes by modeling for me what it means to finish well. But watching them navigate end-of-life realities also sparked my deepest fears: the fear of being incapacitated, of being imprecise, or of being a lesser version of myself because of physical or mental disability.

I experienced this reality for three years recently. Congenital defects in the bones of my legs along with a car accident resulted in multiple surgeries over a three-year time frame. During this time, I was either in a wheelchair or required the use of crutches or a cane. Pain was an unwelcome companion by day and the monster under the bed by night. I was unsure if I would walk without assistance and pain.

Disability can also be considered a relative term. At any given moment on any given day, we might feel less able or more able than . . .

whom, what, when? If I compare my current self to my younger self, then yes, it is true that I can no longer run as fast, jump rope as well, or play basketball as I once did. No doubt my younger self would view my current self's diminished physical capacity and perhaps feel sadness. But I can now look back with fondness and gladness, not mourning. My older self has developed other important abilities.

I remember fondly my mountaintop memories, including hiking Kilimanjaro twice, climbing in New Zealand, and skiing in Colorado. I also realize this book came from my forced rest and disability. I was forced to flex and adapt. I have seen God's intimate work in my life during previous difficult seasons and through learning to surrender.

Surrendering benefits us in all paradigm shifts, but especially our last one. Knowing when to surrender and when to fight is found in the simplicity of the Serenity Prayer:

> *O God and Heavenly Father grant to us the serenity of mind to accept that which cannot be changed, courage to change that which can be changed, and wisdom to know the one from the other through Jesus Christ, our Lord, Amen.*[7]

I realize that I may one day have some sort of illness or accident that leaves me fully incapacitated and bedbound. (I could also die in a plane crash next week.) My point is that it is futile to dread this possible paradigm shift from chronic to disability. Instead, focus on what you *can* do.

An Unexpected Ending

Such was a lesson I learned from Michael. He was in his forties and on dialysis for kidney failure. He lived in constant dread. He worried incessantly about the day when dialysis would no longer be an option for him. He was on the kidney transplant list and spent his days and nights feverishly checking his placement. While he fretted and stressed, his life rambled out of control. He gained weight and worked less, taking jobs farther and farther from home. He would frequently complain, "This stress is killing me!"

He was wrong. On an early morning commute to work, he fell asleep and drifted into the path of an eighteen-wheeler. He died instantaneously. He had spent the preceding two years worrying about a future he would never see.

This tragic story reminds us that, as with most situations in life, perspective is everything. We cannot always choose our next chapters in life. We can choose how we prepare for them and live through them.

It also reminds us that sometimes death arrives like a slow-moving steam engine whose whistle can be heard long before we see it, and sometimes death arrives like an eighteen-wheeler at maximum speed. We don't know which will be ours. The very essence of being human is to be limited by time. Understanding this principle will help us prepare for either ending. It will also give us a greater appreciation for this day which we have been given.

If your suffering feels intolerable and you struggle to see or feel anything beyond it, there is hope through anticipating heaven. It will set your mind free even when your body is declining, transitioning through one paradigm shift after another.

The last time I saw Mr. C was in the hospital cafeteria two months before I transferred to another hospital. He was having lunch with a friend who also had a portable oxygen tank at his feet. They were old golfing buddies who had reconnected at pulmonary rehabilitation.

Mr. C was seeing a palliative care physician and reported he was able to get out more, which made him feel better. He looked better and was able to speak in full sentences. He shared pictures of his new grandson; he was a proud grandpa, just happy to be alive. I smiled as I walked away. I knew that feeling.

Until We Meet Again

It was time to discharge Mrs. R so she could enjoy some final beach time. During her brief hospital stay, she and her husband had shared so much of their wisdom. Their lives had been interrupted, yet she exuded a peace beyond human understanding.

Before she and her husband left, I prayed for her and for the fulfillment of her final wishes. I concluded with the phrase "until we meet again," the three of us believing fervently that we *would* meet again, though probably not in this life. We hugged, and I walked them out of the hospital.

Two years passed, and my husband and I happened to be visiting a nearby church. As we were leaving, I noticed a man who looked familiar sitting alone in the back row. It was Mr. R! We hugged like long-lost friends. He told us he was driving south to the community where he planned to settle, and he had decided in the spur of the moment to stop in for services. Then he told us how Mrs. R had fulfilled her final dreams before dying peacefully at home. He missed her greatly, he said, but also anticipated their reunion.

When I am asked about my confidence in heaven that leads to my anticipation, I think of stories like Mr. and Mrs. R's. I simply state, "I anticipate heaven and *know that I know that I know* because of the evidence."

What are the odds that I cared for the wife of a man who two years later happened to be traveling from Indiana to Hilton Head and we both visited the same church on the same day? Perhaps there is a number, though statistically improbable. Still, I can give personal testimony of God's intimate presence in the improbable, if not impossible.

In medicine, we look at the evidence to determine a diagnosis. In faith, we can look at the evidence to determine the truth of God's inerrant Word, the Bible.

Change is the only constant as we journey through life. As we experience these paradigm shifts from acute to chronic, chronic to disability, and our final paradigm shift, our body's mutability is evident. Our mind adjusts as it endures the unwinding of life. But God's Word never changes, and his faithfulness has a way of surprising us with his mysterious and improbable ways.

> *Let us hold fast the confession of our hope without wavering, for He who promised is faithful.*
>
> HEBREWS 10:23

nine

THE FINAL PARADIGM SHIFT: "WOW, THIS IS IT!"

All my empty dreams suddenly lost their charm
and my heart began to throb with a bewildering
passion for the wisdom of eternal truth.

ST. AUGUSTINE

Bert was a doctor's doctor, the one other physicians consulted when they were ill. He practiced cutting-edge surgery and taught at a prestigious university. When I first met him and his beautiful wife, Christine, through a shared ministry, Bert was four years into his brave battle with amyotrophic lateral sclerosis—more commonly known as ALS or Lou Gehrig's disease.

Most have known someone with ALS or are at least aware of "The Ice Bucket Challenge," a magnificent fundraiser on social media for ALS research. Most also know that ALS is the last disease they would want to have.

I loved Bert from the moment I met him. He had a brace on his arm and was struggling to walk. His body was failing him, but as is the case with ALS, his brilliant mind was unaffected. We sat directly across from each other at a table that was filled with just-met friends focused on ministry, and I was thankful to hear his voice.

He was funny, engaging, authentic, in love with life and with his wife. Bert was a Renaissance man who was dying. He was a highly skilled surgeon who had lost the ability to use his hands. Imagine having your great passion and purpose taken from you. Each little loss of mobility, ability, or agility was like a small death along the journey to big death.

Bert shared a story with me that night about a dinner held at the same restaurant a few weeks prior. After going to dinner with friends, Bert shuffled over (alone) to look at a neighbor's new boat.

I leaned in closer to hear him say,

> I tripped and fell headfirst into the water. At that time, I had a *little* more strength in my arms than I do now. However, as I struggled in the dark to come up for air, I knew I didn't have enough strength to pull myself up onto the dock. Christine had gone inside, thinking I was right behind her. I thought, *Wow, this is it!*
>
> You can't imagine all the thoughts that ran through my mind. Thankfully, one of them was to put my legs down and quit struggling to swim. So I did. Do you know what? It was low tide. I could stand up! I was able to walk to the steps and make my way out of the water.

He gave a little chuckle, the memory softening the terror he must have felt that night.

Sometimes we fight so hard to swim when all we really need to do is stand up. Still, there are times when, rather than fighting to swim or standing up, it is best to lie down and float with the current. This is the final paradigm shift: to go with the flow.

As I came to know Bert's humor, he would probably also quip that lesson number two is never, ever, *ever* take a walk by the water alone if your legs are a little wobbly. Bert could always crack a joke, even in the grimmest of times.

The River of Life

There will come a time in a patient's journey when treatments fail or become intolerable. When life's end is near, often patients know it before anyone else, even if they choose not to say it. Some may not speak of it because they hope they are wrong. Others don't want to hurt their loved ones with the reality of death's approach. Yet the body cannot hide what the mind is hesitant to acknowledge.

My encouragement is to choose transparency if you are in this season. Authentically sharing each emotion you experience will prepare you for a time when you may no longer be able to share. Share with at least one or two others the deep things you are thinking, feeling, and experiencing. This helps you float rather than struggle to swim.

Your soul yearns so intently for what lies ahead that your mind and heart separate from what lies behind. You prepare to leave the land of the dying to enter the land of the living. Between the two is the River of Life. It is God's flowing grace through his Son, Jesus Christ. The gentle current will bring you home. The book of Revelation speaks of such a river:

> [The angel] showed me a pure river of water of life, clear as crystal, proceeding from the throne of God and of the Lamb. In the middle of its street, and on either side of the river, was the tree of life, which bore twelve fruits, each tree yielding its fruit every month. The leaves of the tree were for the healing of the nations. (22:1–2)

We can choose to step into the flow of God's grace. Caregivers, pay close attention to the changing emotions that occur in the dying patient. We must choose our loved one's needs over our own breaking hearts. Navigating the final paradigm shift well requires contemplative conversations. Ask thoughtful questions, and gently encourage your loved one to talk about important things:

- "What are your goals?"
- "What are your biggest fears?"
- "What worries you?"
- "What brings you comfort?"
- "What are your hopes?"
- "What does a good day look like to you?"
- "What keeps you from sleeping?"
- "What do you need today if tomorrow doesn't come?"

When I witness the final season approach, I tell patients, "It's time to consider a change in how we best care for you. Our perspective until now has been doing everything within our power to help you live *longer.* Now we shift to doing everything we can to help you live *better.* This focus will last until your final breath. We are not promised tomorrow, but for however many tomorrows you have left, we want to help you with suffering. I want to answer your questions, and I want to make sure you know you are not alone."

For patients, families, and healthcare proxies, I add the following: "My faith comforts me with the truth that while we can't control how many days of life we get, we *can* always choose how we will live those days." I find this simple statement brings a visible sigh of relief as families make decisions regarding level of care.

An example of this transition would be a hospitalized patient who has failed all therapies. He or she is a Do Not Resuscitate on arrival, and the decision is whether to choose "comfort care only." I always support the patient if this decision is affirmative. If the patient is unable to speak for themselves, the family or healthcare proxy can feel like they are giving up if they are making the decision. A well-written ACP will guide these decisions. Inevitably, someone makes a choice.

As a person of faith, I believe we are the beloved creatures of an intelligent, all-powerful God. I see no contradiction between the principles and facts of science and the idea that an all-knowing Creator would know the exact number of my days.

> So teach us to number our days,
> That we may gain a heart of wisdom. (Psalm 90:12)

My faith gives me both peace and confidence to comfort patients and family members as they walk through this final paradigm shift. Regardless of my patients' and their families' faith, they tend to find comfort in *my* faith. I believe that, with their decisions, they are not taking or adding a day in the life of the patient. God already decided the number of his or her days. But they, and we, are deciding what each day will look like as the end approaches.

Making the Hospice Decision

Patients and families need clinicians who will guide them in decision-making. They don't need someone to lead them (make decisions for them), and they don't need someone to follow them (force them to make all the decisions). The balanced approach is called *participatory decision-making.* An example of this would be noncurative chemotherapy and its associated side effects versus palliative care or hospice care. The clinician would adequately explain each option and allow the patient and their loved ones to take time and make an informed decision.

You can request from your doctor that he or she guide you in participatory decision-making. You can also guide your doctor with the question, "If this were your loved one, what would you do?"

One of the most crucial decision-making points is determining when hospice is needed. Unfortunately, in the continuum of care across multiple clinical sites, discussions about hospice are often not had or had late.

Hospice is traditionally recommended for those not expecting to survive longer than six months. But at the time of this writing, statistics reveal 50 percent of patients are enrolled in hospice for eighteen days or less. Seventy-five percent are enrolled for eighty-four days or less.[1]

The concept of hospice was introduced in the 1960s by Dame Cicely Saunders. In her East London Catholic clinic, Dr. Saunders introduced the concept of caring for the dying patient's multiple sources of pain. This included physical pain, existential disquiet, and spiritual pain.[2]

It is important to understand the various services available through hospice care. In the United States, this currently includes bereavement care for up to thirteen months for the family of the patient *who dies while under hospice care.* I emphasize the latter half of this sentence because this benefit only applies to families of the deceased who was enrolled in hospice at the time of death.

QUESTIONS TO ASK WHEN CHOOSING HOSPICE CARE

I recommend the following questions and considerations before evaluating hospices in your area if in the United States:[3]

- Confirm the hospice provides Medicare services. The Department of Health and Human Services regulates service providers and locations with minimum standard requirements. The website www.medicare.gov has a search bar for identifying clinical locations with quality metrics assigned to each location.
- In the United States, the website of hospice care's governing board, the National Hospice and Palliative Care Organization (NHPCO), www.nhpco.org, has tremendous information including identifying hospices in your area. The website www.caringinfo.org is a division of NHPCO and also provides valuable resources.
- The National Hospice and Palliative Care Organization (NHPCO) recommends two accrediting agencies in addition to Medicare. They are the Joint Commission and Community Health Accreditation Program. Their

websites are www.jointcommission.org and www.chapinc.org. Choose a hospice that has been accredited.
- Does the provider site offer palliative care services for chronic medical conditions in addition to hospice care?
- Does the service have a volunteer program to assist families in caregiving?
- Are after-hours visits or phone calls available?
- How frequently does the hospice nurse visit?
- Is the hospice physician allowed to prescribe any medication for symptom relief? This is an important question to confirm that medications are prescribed based on effectiveness and not cost.
- What support is available for family and caregivers?
- Will your primary care physician continue to have a role in care?
- What services are included to provide comfort for the patient?
- Does the hospice provide for short inpatient hospital stays if symptom management cannot be achieved at home?
- What locations are available for hospice care?
- Can patients receive therapeutic care for pain, such as radiation, while enrolled in the hospice program?
- Is the hospice a faith-based nonprofit? If so, which faith?

My prayer is that you as the patient and you as a loved one find the courage to talk to your clinicians about hospice before it is needed. This may be the simple request that you want to be notified if hospice should be a consideration based upon your clinical condition. The earlier discussion does not hasten death. It does not mean that you are "giving up." It means you want to be proactive in understanding your disease and clinical condition at any given time.

For families and loved ones of a dying patient, the decision can be complicated. What do you do if not everyone agrees on what is right for the patient? One of my friends went through that situation.

She Chose Love

Sara and I meet once per month via a video platform to discuss business. We also have become friends with a shared love of the Lord, love of family, and understanding of the value of purpose. God's love and care have brought us together.

We often share stories of our lives, and on this day we discussed her mother's death from cancer two years prior. Sara teared up at the mention of her mother. I noticed she rubbed her hands, hunching her shoulders forward. In that moment, she looked like a young girl.

I learned more about her mother's death. Sara told me sometimes her mother's passing felt raw, fresh. Other times, it appeared as a faded scar. Her grief would never go away and yet it was changing—it was becoming a reminder of the battle their family went through.

We discussed how difficult it was near the end. The evidence was clear. Her mother's death was imminent. Her sallow skin appeared translucent without the body's protective layer of fat. Both chemotherapy and terminal illness had taken their toll on this once-vibrant woman. Sara didn't know which had caused the final decline. She and her siblings did know that chemotherapy was no longer working. What once was hope now brought only dread. They felt she should stop.

Can you imagine the internal conflict Sara and her siblings must have felt to have come to this conclusion? Of course, they didn't want to lose their mother, yet they must have felt grief as if it had already occurred, along with the unforgettable burden of seeing their mother suffering. This was a fate worse than death.

Their mother chose the path of continuing the treatments. Their father, in his grief, couldn't envision a clear path forward. And so it was. A mother was fighting for what was not to be, and a family was looking for someone, anyone, to guide them in this complex dying journey. They felt alone despite being surrounded by many. In the end, a choice for hospice care was made. She died the next day.

Sara's family didn't believe that hospice killed their beloved mother. But I have seen time and again where hospice was called too late, and the timing coincided with the tragedy of death. Hurting family members blindly blame an institution designed to bring comfort for the death of a loved one. It becomes embedded in their complex grief. It is a deep and pervasive pain unsubstantiated by truth.

So what should you do if you find yourself in a circumstance similar to the one I described? Listen to the patient, who determines the path. But it is helpful to understand the motivation for the path he or she chooses.

Dying patients face extraordinary emotional challenges as they navigate their own feelings and those of the ones they love. They may feel fear, regret, grief, or responsibility.

Regret is often centered on what cannot be changed in the final months. People long for a way to reverse regrets with just a little more time. They are grieving their own death. They feel fear. They prefer holding on to the fragile life they have rather than the loss they can expect.

Yet, in my experience, the dying also feel a sense of responsibility toward those they are leaving behind. Patients know when death is inevitable. They sense the night approaching. But they struggle on, fueled by love. They cannot imagine those around them without them. Therefore, they struggle—because they love.

In Sara's case, allowing her mother to give her love sacrificially by a will to fight was a gift. She chose suffering to the end so that her family could know she fought to be by their side until God called her home. That day, Sara cried the tears of one deeply loved and deeply grieving.

Patients always have the final say in all matters concerning them. Getting to the core of why patients make a decision will bring clarity for the path forward. It may also make the terrible . . . bearable.

COMFORT ME

If you are the patient reading these statements, consider which ones are applicable to you, and perhaps add more of your own. Create your unique list of how you wish to be comforted and give it to doctors, family members, or caregivers who will be there when you need them most.

If you are a loved one, family, friend, or caregiver for the one who is dying, review this list with the patient. Help them describe what comforts they need. Help facilitate meeting these needs.

The following statements are written from the patient's

perspective and are meant to be a glimpse of how love is given and received at the end of life. Some of these words are paraphrased from Christian patients I have known, some are from my own imagination of how I would like to be treated at my life's end, and some are from others who work with and care for the dying. Perhaps they will help you put into words what seems difficult or help you care for a loved one when you don't know how to comfort them.

- "Nurse, loved one, my body is forsaking me. Please treat me with dignity as you would want to be treated."
- "Family and friends, I do not want to be a burden. As my body weakens, I don't know how not to be. I pray you understand."
- "Loved ones, I cannot face the reality of death all day every day. If I need to talk about normal things, make a joke, or tell a story about the crazy neighbor next door, please know this is a valuable if short distraction from my preparations for death."
- "Loved ones, the little things bring me joy now. So many things I took for granted along the way are like treasures to me now."
- "Trusted advisers, proxies, those I'm leaving behind, help me to get my affairs in order. I lie awake thinking about all I should have done but cannot do now, at least not without help. It is okay. In fact, I want you to bring up these things. As hard as it is, as awkward as it feels, talk to me about my funeral."

- "Family and friends, I worry about my children, my elderly parents who will survive me, or my adult disabled child whom I have been caring for. I would love to have solutions to these deep worries before I go. Will you help me think through and talk through these matters?"
- "Friends and loved ones, sometimes I may feel like talking and sometimes I may need you to just sit with me. For the record, I *do* appreciate you coming and showing you care."
- "Loved ones, allow me to express my sorrow. I am preparing for my losses. Listen to me, hold my hand, be still. And it is okay if you cry with me."
- "Everyone, I have failures, regrets, and hurts I still carry. If I bring up such things, will you listen to my concerns? I don't need a solution from you. I'm merely hoping to lay these things down, forgive, and find forgiveness before I rest. Let me know that my life had meaning, value, and purpose, even in (or especially in) my final hours."
- "Those closest to me, let me know that *in your grief*, you will one day be okay. I know you might not *feel* okay for a long time, but you will take care of yourself. I know you will miss me, yet one day you will be okay, and then perhaps someday, you'll even feel okay. This will give me peace."
- "Caregivers, I will not feel like eating at times, and not at all near the end. I know that you mean well, but please do not pressure me to eat."
- "Caregivers, when my lips are dry or my mouth is parched, small sips of water or a mouth sponge dipped in cold water will ease this suffering."

- "Caregivers, if you hear a rattle in my chest, know that this is normal as my time is near. If I appear uncomfortable, please give me the medicine that helps me rest."
- "Caregivers, I may experience a burst of energy in my final days or hours. Help me to accomplish what I try to do while protecting me from falling."
- "Those who share my faith, whatever my guilt or shame, help me remember grace through Jesus Christ. I must fully understand the cost Jesus paid on the cross for my guilt and shame. To carry these emotions to my ending would diminish the price that was paid *for me*."
- "Everyone, as days turn to hours, I may talk to those who have gone before me. I may speak of traveling. I may see the heaven I have anticipated become visually real. I may use words that seem nonsensical, yet they are the words I must use to describe something I have yet to see. I am comforted by what I feel and see. It is important that you accept and validate what I am telling you. Please don't challenge or argue with my musings."[4]
- "Everyone, as days turn to hours, I may also feel fear, anger, agitation, and despair. I may appear restless and try to climb out of bed. I cannot sleep, for fear that when I do, the frightening things I see may cover me. I am not comforted. I am *terminally restless.*[5] Please make sure that my nurse knows and that there is not a physical cause or a medication cause for my restless state. Please don't let me suffer now.

  "I may be restless from my thoughts of lacking closure.

I may need to hear the voice of a loved one or the words, 'I forgive you.' Consider these if I struggle near the end.

"Perhaps this dread which makes me restless is my rejection of grace. You may mourn my lack of faith. I now mourn it too. My soul is anguished as time draws near. Pray that the truth I rejected may be revealed even in my final hour."

- "Those who share my faith, perhaps my faith has been a guiding star on my horizon. Sometimes it seemed so clear, so close, I could physically touch it. Sometimes it was obscured by cloudy nights and frightening storms. Now, as death approaches, its warm light envelops my soul. I don't need to hold it in my arms to know that its presence has not changed. I know my perspective has changed. Remember this: clouds and storms will come and go, but the guiding star remains the same."
- "Loved ones, when I am ready to depart this life, please let me go. Please do not make me feel guilty for leaving. I must detach in my final hours to prepare for my final breath. This process will be gradual, and I may no longer speak. Do not be alarmed; this is normal."
- "Loved ones, when my eyes are closed and I no longer wake and interact, I can still sense your presence. Thank you for being here. I can still hear, and as I am anticipating heaven, would you help me worship my way home? Read Scripture, play worship music, and pray with me. I am looking toward the Savior, and he is calling me home."

Nearing the End

As time draws short in our lives, we have all our senses, our thoughts, our emotions, our heart focused on what is to come. During the last two weeks of life, we see a subtle shift as one begins to separate from their rooted present to their eternal home. In their final hours, patients may experience *near death awareness* (NDA).[6]

NDA is separate from death awareness. The latter is a conscious process of living life with a healthy perspective of human mortality. There are ways to demystify death through discussion and education. Examples are identified at www.theconversationproject.org and www.deathcafe.com. This is a healthy form of death awareness.

NDA, however, is witnessed during some death vigils. The common threads of NDA are emotional comfort and spiritual transformation for the patient. Experiences described include:

- Communicating with or experiencing the presence of someone who is not alive
- Preparing for travel or a change
- Describing a place they can visualize in another realm (for example, heaven)
- Knowing when death will occur[7]

A study of deathbed communications revealed that deaths including NDA were calmer and more peaceful than those in which it was not present.[8] A patient may begin talking to loved ones who are deceased. My friend Ron's final two words, "Jesus, Jesus!" speak to his faith in how the Christian will be greeted as the soul departs the body.

To the degree family members understand and accept NDA,

they are also comforted. Unlike a hallucination, which can occur with delirium at the end of life and may be identified as terminal restlessness, NDA is reported with detailed clarity and is comforting rather than distressing.

Terminal restlessness is the opposite experience for dying patients and their families. As a Christian physician, when I witness terminal restlessness, I always evaluate the three potential causes for its origin.

- Is there an underlying physical issue such as pain, urinary retention, disease, or medication effect causing the restlessness?
- Is there a psychosocial cause for restlessness? For example, is a family member not present who the dying patient needs to hear from, or does the patient need to ask forgiveness from someone not present?
- Is there a spiritual cause for despair resulting in restlessness at the end of life?

Families must also consider these possibilities as they care for their loved one and know when to ask for clinical help and when to ask for spiritual help. Clinical help can be found by calling the hospice nurse. Have a plan for who would be called if you sense a spiritual need. Is it a pastor, priest, rabbi, friend, or trusted relative?

"I See Heaven"

In the Bible, we read about Stephen, an early follower of Jesus Christ. The religious leaders of the day hated him for it. He would not be silenced and was stoned to death on account of his faith. I believe Scripture depicts Stephen's NDA and the merging of two worlds:

> [Stephen], being full of the Holy Spirit, gazed into heaven and saw the glory of God, and Jesus standing at the right hand of God, and said, "Look! I see the heavens opened and the Son of Man standing at the right hand of God!"
>
> Then [the leaders] cried out with a loud voice, stopped their ears, and ran at him with one accord; and they cast him out of the city and stoned him. And the witnesses laid down their clothes at the feet of a young man named Saul. And they stoned Stephen as he was calling on God and saying, "Lord Jesus, receive my spirit." Then he knelt down and cried out with a loud voice, "Lord, do not charge them with this sin." And when he had said this, he fell asleep. (Acts 7:55–60)

Whether you are the patient or the family member reading this Scripture passage, how does it make you feel? Stephen didn't have an opportunity to develop his unique list of "comfort me" statements. And for some of us, our deaths will also arrive suddenly. But God, in his mercy, was Stephen's comforter by revealing the heaven he anticipated and would enter on that day. God can be our comforter when we trust in him.

Living with the End in Mind

Remember my dear friend Bert from the beginning of this chapter? ALS continued to take from his physical body. But he and his wife had learned to *live with the end in mind.* They planned for choices long before they ever needed them. He neared the end of his life and rested in the gentle current which delivered him home.

Bert served the Lord with his life, dying, and death. He has lost that which he could not keep and gained that which he could not lose. I look forward to seeing him in his heavenly body. It is one of the multitude of reasons I anticipate heaven.

The beauty of this final paradigm shift in your physical body is it precedes the moment when you will think, like Bert did, *Wow, this is it!* I pray your next thought will be these verses:

> *For to me, to live is Christ, and to die is gain.*
> PHILIPPIANS 1:21
>
> *Don't let your hearts be troubled. Trust in God, and trust also in me [Jesus].*
> JOHN 14:1 NLT

ten

THE POWER OF PRAYER IN GOD'S SOVEREIGN CARE

I pray because I can't help myself. I pray because I'm helpless. I pray because the need flows out of me all the time, waking and sleeping. It doesn't change God. It changes me.

C. S. LEWIS

Paul and Debbie endured one of life's greatest tragedies—the death of their four-year-old daughter, Morgan. Understandably, they battled deep pain and anger. But unlike many couples whose marriages disintegrate in the traumatic aftermath of losing a child, Paul and Debbie's marriage somehow survived. They knew they were stronger together rather than apart. They still had a son to raise.

Debbie was a pillar of strength and faith. She was a steady influence in Paul's life as he raged at a God who would take his baby girl. Paul's journey to faith was long and arduous, but, once there, he embraced it fully. He became a flame, a person everyone wanted to be near just to feel the warmth. He was truly larger-than-life. His faith in Jesus Christ and his anticipation of heaven gave him a perspective that was powerful to those with whom he shared his faith.

Debbie called me one Saturday morning while I was working. She said that Paul had a cut on his arm that appeared to be infected. She reported a redness surrounding it and extending down his arm. While refusing to have the cut checked, Paul had become weak and lethargic. He was not eating. I recommended Debbie call 911, and I assured her that I would evaluate Paul in the ER.

When he came in, my heart sank. He was a shell of the man I knew. His cheeks were gaunt, his lips were cracked, his skin was a yellowish-green, and his eyes were yellow from jaundice. He recognized me but showed symptoms consistent with delirium. His vitals were abnormal, and our initial working diagnosis was "sepsis with shock with suspected skin source."

The definition of *sepsis* is "the body's overwhelming and life-threatening response to infection that can lead to tissue damage, organ failure, and death."[1] It is your body's overactive and toxic response to an infection. Like strokes or heart attacks, sepsis is a medical emergency that requires rapid diagnosis and treatment. It is serious. It can strike young or old, and mortality rates can be high if not caught early.

We started Paul on antibiotics and fluids to improve his blood pressure while we waited for his lab work to return. Debbie stood by nervously as her teenage and young adult children arrived. They were anxious to know more about their dad. I began to get results from his initial laboratory studies, and my worst fears were confirmed. Paul had sepsis, and the infection was causing his organs to fail. In addition to his altered mental status, tests showed severe liver damage and acute kidney failure.

Debbie and her children stood in shock as they attempted to process the severity of Paul's condition. I could see the fear in Debbie's eyes. She was a woman who was well acquainted with loss. When I, her trusted "doctor friend," recommended a medical university two hours away, she did not second-guess my decision.

We stabilized Paul at our small hospital and transferred him to the regional medical university. In that new environment, Debbie no longer had a physician friend on staff to call. This is the experience of most patients and their families.

Paul was admitted to one of the specialty ICUs at the university. Initially he showed some improvement following surgery on his arm and treatment of the secondary effects of sepsis. However, a few nights after his admission, we received a call that his heart had stopped, and a code blue had been called. *Code blue* is a universal indicator of a serious cardiac or respiratory event that needs immediate response.

The medical staff were able to resuscitate Paul. His vital signs remained tenuous, and his clinical status was critical and unstable. Doctors shared the grim news with Debbie that her sweetheart may not survive the night.

The Call Tree

I have discovered regardless of hospital or situation, God always has a remnant of his praying people who work in such settings. Ask for them at the hospital, as is your right. You may ask for a Christian chaplain, other Christian services of volunteers that pray, or if there are doctors or nurses who pray for their patients and families. The latter question may be greeted with a blank stare or a genuine answer. Don't let the potential stare keep you from finding the spiritual care. Those working in places where life and death collide on a frequent basis often have profound faith. Even when you don't ask, they are praying.

For my friends Paul and Debbie, an informal call tree for prayer requests was activated. A small group of us drove through the night to be with Debbie. The two-hour ride felt endless, as we did not know what to expect when we arrived. We were weighed down with the somber realization of the fragility of life. But we also believed that faith and hope are powerful. Our group prayed fervently as we drove.

That night, we walked the hallway outside the ICU praying silently and taking turns in Paul's room with Debbie and her children as space allowed. The proximity to death made the ICU's rules about the number of guests in Paul's room less important.

Paul survived the night, but never woke. For two long, hard, sad months, he was on life support. When the machines were slowly withdrawn, he remained in a comatose state. He was transferred back to our hometown hospital so Debbie and her children could return to their home, with one less family member by their side.

Paul's dying was like a candle flame, his life flickering till the last spark faded. It was peaceful. But I considered my patient who told me she was going to have a good death, and I knew Paul had lived anticipating heaven and a reunion with his daughter, Morgan.

It may seem impossible to find good in death. We cannot rely on platitudes or false hopes when prayers seemingly go unanswered. These are the moments when faith is shattered, born, or strengthened. We pray to accept God's will as perfect and that it is a divine mystery.

HOW TO BUILD A CALL TREE

Regardless of health condition, having a call tree and prayer tree is wise. This prepares you for the expected and unexpected. It is especially crucial if you or your loved one has a serious or terminal diagnosis. A call and prayer tree are created in the same manner and may be one and the same depending on your circumstance.

- Considering a crisis, such as Debbie faced, designate one person whom you trust to be the person you or your loved one calls. Designate another person as a backup in the event your primary person is unreachable.
- That person will notify the next two people in your tree, and they will each notify the next two people, and so forth. The concept is to identify the fastest way to relay information and to have people praying in an emergency.
- This system also works to notify those with predetermined roles that they have been activated. For example, one person may notify family, another person may notify schools or employers, and someone else may take care of pets. All of this is initiated with just one call from someone who is with the patient.
- This method of relaying information helps you as the patient or you as the loved one to focus on what is happening in the clinical setting rather than on making multiple calls.

Many things about Paul's death were not (and are not) good. Widowhood is not good. Three kids not having their dad is not good. Saying goodbye to an amazing friend is not good. An empty seat at the dining table is not good.

Yet Paul would have been the first to say he had found great strength and joy in life through his faith. *That* is good. The faith he found after losing a child was inspiring and contagious to others, and that, too, was good. During his last years, Paul had a remarkable way of treating each moment in life as a gift—a memory that can still bring my husband to tears all these years later. That is *really* good.

Paul's big, full life with family and friends, and his hard death in the strange land of hospitals and ICUs, are sobering reminders that we each are granted a finite number of precious moments. Our ending is dependent upon our beginning, our middle, and finally, on how we finish.

God's sovereign care exists even in times when we suffer greatly. I have been taught this valuable lesson through personal suffering, patients' suffering, and stories like Paul's and Debbie's. Though we grieve our circumstances, we can trust our Father God, who walks with us through them.

Preparing Your Soul Through Prayer

We've talked about preparing minds and hearts, and about practical matters as we anticipate the end of life on earth and the beginning of life in heaven. Now let us focus on preparing the soul to go home. The most basic way to do this is through prayer.

Prayer is a powerful gift when we need it most. Suffering may bring us to our knees in prayer. But prayer is also a spiritual practice that benefits us in the absence of a crisis, medical or otherwise. How do we develop a vibrant prayer life?

- Commit to prayer as a practice.
- Create a consistent time and place for prayer.
- Consider prayer a sacred time of communication with the Creator.
- Cultivate bidirectional communication; prayer, as with conversations, should be bidirectional. Give praise, give petition, give gratitude, and then listen. I struggle with the listening. My brain becomes a pinball machine each time I try to keep it still. But with time, I am learning. Remember, this is a practice.
- Call upon the Lord when discernment is needed.
- Cry out to the Lord in times of brokenness.
- Contemplate what Jesus said about how to pray:

> Our Father in heaven,
> Hallowed be Your name.
> Your kingdom come.
> Your will be done
> On earth as it is in heaven.
> Give us this day our daily bread.
> And forgive us our debts,
> As we forgive our debtors.
> And do not lead us into temptation,
> But deliver us from the evil one.
> For Yours is the kingdom and the power and the glory forever.
> Amen. (Matthew 6:9–13)

- Concede that not all prayers are answered in the manner we asked for. If this were true, wouldn't the prayers of a faith-filled child always be answered? Wouldn't the lives of the young be spared based on potential and merit? Jesus revealed this to us in his prayer in the garden of Gethsemane:

> "Father, if it is Your will, take this cup away from Me; nevertheless not My will, but Yours, be done." Then an angel appeared to Him from heaven, strengthening Him. And being in agony, He prayed more earnestly. Then His sweat became like great drops of blood falling down to the ground. (Luke 22:42–44)

The last point is vital to understand. Jesus prayed for a different path to fulfill God's plan. He was strengthened by an angel and still "prayed more earnestly" and his sweat became like drops of blood—actually, *great drops of blood.* His anguish in knowing he would be separated from the Father for the first time revealed his humanity. His unanswered prayer ultimately revealed a gift to humanity that can never be surpassed.

PRAYER AND SCIENCE

Between the late 1990s and 2015, there was great curiosity and debate in the scientific world about the power of prayer with respect to healing. As scientists explored this subject using advanced medical research methods, it became clear that a religious-scientific consensus would never be reached.

Many used the Harvard Prayer Experiment from 2006 as their point of reference.[2] This study's conclusion reported no benefit on healing outcomes for patients who received a specific intercessory prayer and those who did not. Others cited studies that did seem to show *some* health benefits as a result of prayer.

Some scientists believe the problem with such intercessory prayer studies is that it is difficult, if not impossible, to conduct accurate testing. How can researchers adequately measure and monitor how much prayer is being offered on behalf of someone who is sick? How many people are praying? How often are they praying? Where are they praying? Since these factors vary widely from patient to patient (as do patient treatments), the obvious question is, How can the "results" of individuals be meaningfully compared?

Jeff Levin, a social epidemiologist, reviewed sixteen hundred studies that evaluated the correlation between religious and spiritual participation and health. He concluded that, regardless of religious affiliation, disease, health condition, age, sex, race, ethnicity, or nationality, prayer *does* seem to make a positive difference in some cases.[3]

Perhaps, however, the real reason some frown upon such studies is that they consider the subject matter "incompatible with the current view of the physical universe and consciousness."[4] They simply are not open to the possibility of a spiritual reality.

I personally don't see a specific value in the scientific study of prayer outcomes. *Prayer and outcomes are supernatural events.* While the supernatural determines the foundational principles of science, science cannot explain the foundational principles of the supernatural.

And there is a truth no one can refute, as it has been proven repeatedly: there are positive effects of prayer and/or meditation for the patient regardless of their healing outcome. Previous studies have revealed improved physical, psychological, social, and spiritual well-being.[5 6 7 8] Couldn't we all benefit in these areas?

Prayer, Worship, and the Word of God

Meanwhile, what about my friend Debbie? She had lost a child and then her husband. How much grief can one person endure? When I told her I wanted to tell Paul's story in this book and I read to her what I had initially written, I did not mention their daughter's death. Instead, *she* brought it up. She spoke eloquently about how she had managed to find good in tragedy. It deepened her faith and sparked faith in Paul's heart. Debbie considers this her greatest treasure.

Losing their daughter, Morgan, resulted in the births of their two youngest children. Prior to Morgan's death, Debbie and Paul had decided to stop at two children. In fact, a tubal ligation had already been scheduled. Now, whenever she looks at her two youngest children, she also sees her precious Morgan.

Despite her grievous losses, Debbie is living with genuine faith. She is a student of God's Word and worships God in the beauty of his creation and the miracle of her grandchildren she now holds. She understands faith does not exclude her from suffering. Her grief of losing Morgan and Paul is a weight she carries. It reflects her love. But her faith and anticipation of heaven give her spiritual strength that defies gravity. She would be the first to tell you:

> I consider that the sufferings of this present time are not worthy to be compared with the glory which shall be revealed in us. (Romans 8:18)

Prayer, worship, and the Word of God help change fear to anticipation. They help change the unknown to being known.

Why pray through suffering? I can tell you what it means for me as I anticipate heaven.

- Because I pray, I *anticipate* a closer relationship with God.
- Because I pray, I *anticipate* a closer relationship with others.
- Because I pray, I *anticipate* a unique ability to share the gospel of Jesus Christ amid my suffering.
- Because I pray, I *anticipate* that I will be healed.

How can I declare that I will be healed? How can you? We can pray for our physical bodies to be healed. When God chooses to answer our prayers with physical healing, it is called a miracle. But we can also choose to be healed in our souls. The word *sozo* is the Greek word translated as "saved." This word also means "healed."[9]

The only prayer I know that results in a miracle *every single time* is the prayer that results in salvation. It is the prayer of admitting sin, asking Jesus to forgive, and acknowledging his death and resurrection as God's Son and our Savior who reigns over our life.

Christians should pray in faith for a miracle but acknowledge we have already experienced the greatest miracle we will ever witness.

God sent his one and only Son to the cross to bear the fullness of his wrath for you and for me. When God looks at my heart, my thoughts, my actions, he sees Jesus and the cross. I don't know about you, but I *know* I don't deserve that; and I am immensely grateful for this exquisite miracle of redemption.

As you navigate your illness or that of a loved one, please know that I have committed to pray every day while I have breath for God to heal the reader of these words with his perfect eternal healing. Though my friend Paul died in his physical body, his soul was *healed*, and that helps me *know* I will one day see him again.

Physical healing through medicine or even a miracle is still temporary. The physical body will ultimately die. But the soul is eternal. Are you healed in your soul?

> *Have mercy on me, O Lord, for I am weak; O Lord, heal me, for my bones are troubled. My soul also is greatly troubled; But You, O Lord—how long? Return, O Lord, deliver me! Oh, save me for Your mercies' sake!*
>
> PSALM 6:2–4

eleven

HOPE AMID SUFFERING

If there is a meaning in life at all, then there must be a meaning in suffering. Suffering is an ineradicable part of life, even as fate and death. Without suffering and death, human life cannot be complete.

DR. VIKTOR FRANKL

In the previous chapter we discussed prayers and miracles. But what if prayers aren't answered? What if miracles are not received? Is there a possibility of something good to come from the suffering you and your loved ones are experiencing now?

Suffering is real. As we anticipate the end of life on earth, suffering is inevitable. I have walked with those who have experienced every possible kind of suffering. But it wasn't until 2009 and my first medical mission trip that I came to understand atrocious suffering may ultimately lead to *good*. Incessant suffering may lead to fulfilling a God-given purpose. And end-of-life suffering may result in families and communities ushering the dying person home with worship, praise, and confidence. Perhaps that's a miracle of another kind.

Going to Rwanda throughout the years and sharing my family's life with our Rwandan family has changed my perspective on every aspect of life. We've sponsored several children through Africa New Life Ministries and have come to know their families as our family. They've impacted my spiritual life, my family life, and my professional life in medicine. Therefore, I'd like to share three stories from Rwanda that may also comfort your unique suffering as you prepare for the end of life. Perhaps as you read them, their lessons will reveal to you an application in your life as the patient or your life as a loved one. They may reduce avoidable suffering, the suffering of *regrets.*

The Broken Heart of Africa

Imagine traveling back in time to the late 1950s and ascending into the heavens, then looking down on the heart of Africa known as Rwanda. If we could do that, you would see a host of tiny lights flickering faintly across the countryside.

For the record, those are not campfires. They are the embers of a cultural, tribal wildfire that will eventually sweep across the nation. As the conflagration spreads, many families will separate, scattering in every direction and hoping somehow to survive and meet again one day.

This inferno of evil will be fueled for decades by the combustible ingredients of colonialism and identity politics. Greedy leaders who seek power by sowing fear will fan it. Thus, it will only be a matter of time until the nation finds itself in a firestorm of hatred.

If we look closely enough, we might even see the sorrow of

a father standing on a mountain in Uganda looking south at the "Land of a Thousand Hills." This is the place where his children once played freely, a tiny country of 10,169 square miles[1]—and it is now flowing with blood.

In 1993, a peace treaty (or at least a power-sharing agreement) was negotiated between leaders of opposing groups, between the Government of the Republic of Rwanda and the Rwandan Patriotic Front. But on April 6, 1994, a plane carrying the Rwandan president, a Hutu, was shot down. When that happened, all hopes for peace dissipated. Hutu extremist groups like the Interahamwe, which means "Those Who Attack Together," and the Impuzamugambi, which means "Those Who Have the Same Goal," went into overdrive. They spread the vile idea that the Tutsis were not human. They said they were cockroaches to be hunted, stamped out, and annihilated. Dehumanization is always an initial component of genocide.

Through intimidation and fear, the few convinced the many to form murderous packs. These mobs set about killing their Tutsi friends and neighbors. Churches, thought to be places of sanctuary, became like the furnaces of Auschwitz. The longer the killings went on, the darker and more despicable the stories got. Rape. Torture. Dismemberment. Beheadings. All Tutsis would be targeted (and sometimes the Hutus who attempted to protect them). Babies and children, grandmothers and grandfathers, and everyone in between.

By the end of a horrific hundred-day killing spree, over a million Tutsis and those who sympathized with them were murdered by their Hutu neighbors. Meanwhile, the world sat idly by, focused on lesser fires, nearer problems, other things.

Have you seen enough yet?

For the survivors who lost loved ones to these violent acts, perhaps the most challenging yet practical questions begin with the word *how*.

How is it possible to go on with life in the aftermath of such evil? *How* can such trauma and grief be healed? *How* can so much suffering exist in a country the size of the state of Maryland in the United States?

While every death is devastating, for the surviving loved ones of those who die due to the violent acts of others, the trauma is overwhelming. Is it possible for souls shattered by violent deaths to find healing? Is there any way for a bit of beauty to come out of tragedy? Can love conquer hate? Is it possible that, even though a violent death cannot be erased or undone, it might somehow be redeemed? Can suffering on this scale teach us anything about our own suffering, which is *very, very, real*?

Blessed

My understanding of how good can be birthed from the unimaginable began when I spent time with a genocide survivor. His name is Blessed.

When I first met Blessed, I noticed the scar above his left eyebrow and recognized its shape. It was like a crescent moon set in the darkness of the night, the shape of a machete's scar that had been stretched by years of growth from child to adult man.

I never ask questions when I see the scars of violence. I do not want to draw attention to memories shrouded in fear. I simply said, "I love your name." In a place where so much pain, horror, and inhumanity took place, names like Blessed, Promise, Peace, and Grace are prevalent. A horrific history of genocide was not forgotten but was replaced with names of life, hope, and healing.

Blessed, like so many others, had a story to share. We walked together with the country's stunning beauty stretched out before us, and he began talking to me. "I love my country, and I love my president," he said. "I am blessed to live here, and mostly I am blessed that I am alive."

"I love your nation too," I replied. "And I'm also grateful to have so many friends here. I love the feeling I get when I step off the plane. For me, it is like coming to my home away from home. This is a place of blessing, and you are Blessed."

He smiled and explained, "My auntie gave me that name when I survived the attack. At first, they thought I was dead. My parents did not survive the genocide. Only my sister and I did."

Joyfully, he continued, "I am an uncle now! My mother and father would be so happy to know this. My auntie laughs all the time that my niece is just like my mother was as a young girl. Even though Queen is only four, she is always trying to be the mother to others."

"Each person I have met here has a history of intense suffering," I said. "I can tell they are still suffering when tears fill their eyes in remembrance. But despite suffering, the most joyful people I know live here. How is that possible?"

He stopped and looked at me. "We have learned how to love again."

"How?" I asked softly. "How did you learn to love again?"

"You must begin with forgiveness. I cannot speak for others, but for me, there was no alternative. I could not live my life until I forgave those who caused death."

I am sure Blessed's parents would be so proud of him. Through the miracle and mystery of forgiveness, he has found the ability to love rather than hate. Out of unspeakable evil, undeniable good has arisen: a generation of children with names like Grace and Peace and Blessed who are agents of love and who want to overcome suffering with love and forgiveness.

Blessed had to choose to forgive, and when he did, he learned how to love. Blessed still suffers from missing his parents, he has frequent headaches, and food is sometimes scarce, but Blessed laughs with his whole body and sings Christian music in Kinyarwanda (the official language of Rwanda). He goes to church on Sundays and Wednesdays and has found work.

Yes, Blessed is blessed, and I hope you read his story closely because he shares a lot with few words. To forgive and to be forgiven are compelling elements of a peaceful ending filled with love.

Patients who reach the end of their lives with fractured personal relationships intensely suffer the loss as time for reconciliation grows short. Peace sometimes carries a cost, which may involve the exchange of *being right* for *being with.* Avoidable suffering begins with tending to relational regrets.

Families and caregivers, if your loved one is experiencing restlessness, consider the possibility that he or she has an unmet need for reconciliation. Make every attempt to fulfill this need for peace.

Pacifique's Dream

Years after my conversation with Blessed, I was in Rwanda again for medical missions and had another conversation I'll never forget. It was 5:30 a.m., and a fellow physician and I had decided to run the distance from our hospital in Kigali, Rwanda, to another hospital in a small community fifteen miles away. We prayed for the conditions in which good doctors worked to provide care for a burgeoning population. This early morning run was our time to pray and reflect on God's creation and his love for the people of Rwanda.

There was a chill in the air. The sun had not yet risen, and I was a little nervous. My friend was a serious runner, and I had not run in many months. What's more, Rwanda's rolling hills presented a daunting challenge to someone who lives at sea level. I was thankful when two more friends joined us. I knew the three natural athletes could run together.

As we set out, a young man dressed in a sweatshirt and long pants was running the same direction as we departed the hospital. The man introduced himself as Pacifique. I settled into his pace, which was in fact more my pace. I waved to my friends to go on ahead. "I'll catch up, and if I don't, pick me up on the ride back."

I love meeting new people, and I especially love hearing someone's story. Stories are treasures to me. However, this story was one of sadness and lost dreams.

"I work now for a company. However, I had a dream to build green farming co-ops so farmers in the villages could find a better way to provide for their families," he said.

"*Had* a dream?" I inquired.

He looked down at our shuffling feet. "My friend and I shared this dream . . . until he died one month ago. This is the first time I have run since his death. We always used to run together. I thought if I couldn't have our dream, at least I could have our run."

He was suffering the pain of loss. He had lost his friend, and he had lost their shared dream.

At first, I had assumed that this chance encounter with Pacifique was so I might have someone to run with at my slow pace. In that moment, however, it became apparent to me that it was orchestrated by God. I needed to encourage my new friend with my own story about dreaming dreams and seeing them realized.

I told him the place where he had joined us in running was

called the Dream Medical Center. It is part of the Africa New Life Dream Center. It was founded by Dr. Charles and Florence Mugisha, my friends and mentors.

Before the clinic was founded, the Dream Center was built on the belief that everyone deserves a chance to dream. It was a place for faith, with a vibrant church and a seminary that trained pastors to serve East Africa and beyond. It was a place for hope, where mothers were taught job skills and discipled. Most important, it was a place for love to be shared with the widows, the orphaned, and the poor.

I told Pacifique that I had to come to his country from halfway around the world to realize my dreams. The big hospital behind us was once only a small dream—the vision for a small medical clinic intended to serve the poor of Rwanda. That dream had been planted in my heart and in the heart of another doctor a decade earlier, after we had spent a week in the area caring for the poor.

We discovered that Dr. Charles had been dreaming about adding a medical clinic to the Dream Center, and our hearts caught fire. A small dream became a *big, reckless* dream—the kind of dream that is bound not by the possible but the limitless, because it was a God-placed dream. I shared my experience in my Christian walk that when God asks me to do a big thing, he reveals his presence by the people he brings to the journey.

I shared with Pacifique that the Dream Medical Center is now considered one of the best in Rwanda. I encouraged him with the truth that our God-sized dreams came to pass despite our weaknesses, and that his dreams did not have to end just because he now dreams alone. God would bring people to help him fulfill the dream.

I must have been out of breath by that point, because our run continued for a few moments in silence. Finally, he said, "Thank you for helping me to see my dream again. It is also a reckless dream. I like that." A few moments later he added, "My friend that I ran with, he was my younger brother."

Why do I share this with you as you confront your own suffering? Because the suffering of regret may be felt in unrealized potential and unmet dreams. Because it reminds me that God places goals and dreams in the hearts of his people. But he almost always uses more than one person to fulfill his plans. If part of your suffering is related to unfinished dreams, unfulfilled purpose, take heart. Your interrupted life can carry on through the lives of your dream-bearers.

If you have breath, God will give you purpose. You or your loved ones may feel that your suffering prevents you from fulfilling God's purposes in your lives. But perhaps you will fulfill them *because* of your suffering. Suffering gives you a stage, and pain becomes a microphone. People *listen.* You may find your purpose in sharing the wisdom you gained from success and failure during your lifetime. It may exist in *communicating your regret* so that those you love will not experience the same.

You may be in your life's last quarter or even overtime, but you are still in the game or God would have called you home.

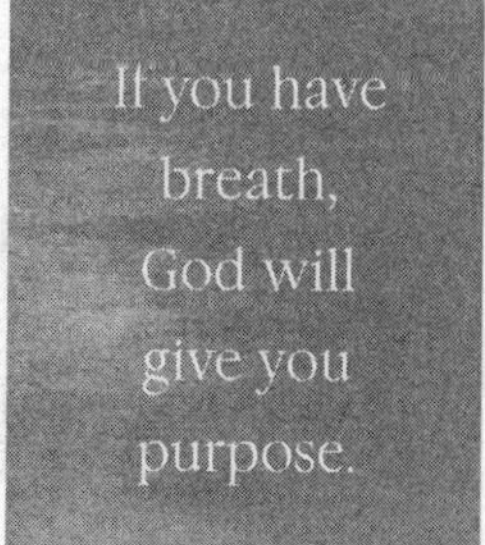
If you have
breath,
God will
give you
purpose.

Remember that God sees and hears you in your suffering. Take courage and turn toward your dream—let yourself "see" it again—and ask God to show you your purpose as you run toward your finish line. Don't fixate on regrets and things you can't change, and don't diminish the life you could still live.

Tom and Kaka: Living While Suffering

A year after my run with Pacifique, I met my friend Tom at his house in Sunzu Village, Rwanda. His house was perched perilously on the side of a mountain overlooking a lake and a volcano. While he could have built this house quickly, he instead chose the slow pace. His neighbors were subsistence farmers who were making a living in the best way they knew how. Poverty was prevalent and suffering was inevitable, even expected.

He employed many for the ten years it took to build this house, a home that could have been built in two. He created a micro-economy in the little village nestled between volcanoes. Tom now hosts visitors from near and far for an incredible organization called Bridge2Rwanda.[2] Heads of state and industry sit at the same table where those from the village break bread.

Though Tom had enjoyed a busy and successful life as an attorney in Southern California, he felt something was missing. He wanted more intentionality in his life. He *needed* to live for a greater purpose. He decided to move to Rwanda and live among the people he had grown to love. This was not a retirement that would consist of lazy days and evening cocktail hours. Tom went to Rwanda with the goal of creating jobs, building schools, and building community centers. He wanted to live a meaningful life, a life of service to others.

One of his daily visits was to a blind widow known as Kaka ("grandmother" in English). When I came to see him, my husband and I and our friends Darrin and Leslie joined him on a visit. We visited the children at the school that morning and then set out on the trek to where she lived.

I remember Kaka sitting on a bench outside her home. Her

home was composed of mud bricks with a corrugated metal roof. I thought about how loud it must be when it rains. The rainy season in Rwanda brings downpours, not gentle showers.

Kaka's shoulders were draped in a red sweater, perhaps a gift from a previous visitor. Her hands, gnarled with age, held an equally gnarled cane. She broke into a smile as she heard us approaching on the steep, single-person dirt path etched into the mountainside by countless bare feet. Tom's friendly greeting elicited raucous laughter.

The two hugged as the old friends they were, and she hugged the rest of us warmly as Tom poured her a glass of fermented milk and placed it in her hands. She loved this Rwandan version of buttermilk. She drank it in one gulp and then laughed as she spoke rapidly in Kinyarwanda. She thanked Tom for the milk and the other provisions he had brought up the mountain. He handed her son the soap, cooking oil, and rice.

Kaka shared her bench with me, and I couldn't help but put my arm around her bony shoulders. She laughed in delight at having visitors. I could feel her insides rattle. At the time, Kaka was believed to be somewhere north of ninety years old. She was living a good life and yet had incessant suffering from arthritis pain exacerbated by the changing weather patterns. She had survived the genocide in which many of her family members had been killed. She had lived through darkness but had the light of Jesus within her. She wore her suffering in silence and gave glory to God for each day.

Everyone in the village knew Kaka. She was "grandmother" to all. Despite her suffering, she brought laughter, love, and joy to those who visited. During one of the rainy seasons, she became ill. Many came to visit and help her son as her time of suffering was about to end. They became her hospice.

I can't imagine the life Kaka lived and the atrocities she experienced. Yet, despite pain, an inability to walk very far, and blindness, her service to the Lord was greeting those with a smile that brought joy to your heart. It was a simple but powerful calling. She had a quiet death—fell asleep, and didn't wake up. Her work was done.

Kaka lived anticipating heaven, and I can only imagine when she saw his glory for the first time. I smile at the thought of her eternal body. I imagine her blind eyes seeing, and the first person she sees is her beloved Savior. Her gnarled physical body is replaced with her glorious heavenly body. I hope her laugh remains unchanged.

Two years after my visit, Tom had a major hemorrhage in his brain. His hold on life was tenuous. He shouldn't have survived. He scarcely did. As soon as he was able, he returned to his life's purpose despite his suffering, or perhaps because of it.

Tom and Kaka both experienced suffering while giving and receiving love with great joy. I have yet to meet a person who confronts his or her own mortality and regrets that more hours were not spent on work, or more wealth gained. Regrets are found in the days without love.

In the words of Mother Teresa, "In this life we cannot do great things. We can only do small things with great love."[3] Tom and Kaka shared this simple message. I hope their stories remind you that even in suffering, you can too.

Perspective Through Suffering

In Rwanda, I have met many who have suffered greatly. I've met those who suffer from physical conditions who may not have the same access to treatments that we do. I've met those who suffer as they work from dusk to dawn to provide for their families and may feel like they always fall just short. I've met perpetrators of the genocide who have been forgiven by everyone, including our Father, but cannot forgive themselves.

Despite the immensity of suffering that exists here, or perhaps as a result, I've seen a deep, abiding dependence on Jesus Christ. The people of Rwanda witnessed the depth and breadth of evil possible in the heart of humanity. This nation cried out to God in their pain. Suffering still exists, but it ignites their love of God and gratitude for his presence. Their prayers are centered on worship, praise, and gratefulness.

For those in Rwanda, the patients I've described in this book, and the thousands of others who have had a suffering journey, including myself, *perspective* makes the difference. I know there will be days when your suffering may seem intolerable. There will also be days when you find goodness despite it.

Don't let your suffering be the result of regrets that can still be changed. And for those that can't, place them at the foot of the cross. Your suffering can be a catalyst for growth. It can result in a deeper relationship with God as you become dependent on his strength, not yours. This dependency allows you to comfort others as God comforts you:

> Blessed be the God and Father of our Lord Jesus Christ, the Father of mercies and God of all comfort, who comforts us in all our tribulation, that we may be able to comfort those who are in any trouble, with the comfort with which we ourselves are comforted by God. (2 Corinthians 1:3–4)

The apostle Paul suffered greatly as he spread the good news. Yet he considered it nothing in comparison to the coming glory. He *anticipated heaven*!

> *For I consider that the sufferings of this present time are not worthy to be compared with the glory which shall be revealed in us.*
>
> ROMANS 8:18

twelve

THE MOST IMPORTANT PREPARATION

There is a place of quiet rest, near to the heart of God.
CLELAND MCAFEE

Billy Graham was one of the greatest evangelists in history. He asked this question with the power and authority of a man filled with the Holy Spirit and on a holy mission: "Are *you* prepared to die?"

That's a question that hits us in all its urgency. We have spent the preceding chapters together preparing you as the patient for the first time you hear the diagnosis, for life with a serious diagnosis, and for how to plan for the hard hard in the dying process.

You have met those who experienced a journey that may be like yours or those with unexpected outcomes through miracles. I have written for you as the patient or you as a loved one. Through the chapters I pray that you felt God's presence and learned how to *anticipate heaven* amid your suffering with prayer and belief.

But when Billy Graham asked "Are you prepared to die?" he wasn't asking about any of these preparations with which you are now equipped. He was asking, "Is your soul prepared to die?" Then he would share the gospel of Jesus Christ.

His sermons were often followed by phrases like this: *If you are not sure, or if you don't have a day and time defined, then come forward and let's make this your defining moment!*

If you have read this book thus far and found value in the practical content but not so much in the "religious" parts, would you please stay with me in this chapter? The word *religion* can bring thoughts of division, hypocrisy, and intolerance. But faith—deep, abiding faith—brings unity, transparency, and love. Isn't that worth seeking?

Or if you have read this book thus far, and the stories and scriptures have given you encouragement and strengthened your faith, may I ask you to do something? Remember the moment or season when you met Jesus and you *believed*. It will remind you of your first love and refresh you in this moment. If you write it down, it will bring peace, joy, and hope for those you may leave behind.

This chapter is the most important preparation you need to make, whether you are a patient or not.

Are you prepared to die?

A Spiritual Before and After

Let me briefly share the story of a man who was not prepared to die and lived to tell about it. He is my husband, Scott.

Scott knew Jesus from the religion he had experienced as a child. But that same religion resulted in him rejecting Jesus as Lord and Savior. He knew personally the experience of sitting in pews on Sunday with those who lived an entirely different life every other day of the week. He experienced the pain of a broken home as so many of us do. But his pain became entwined with the contradiction of his family in church versus at home.

He was too young to discern the human condition from human conditioning associated with rules of religion. He may have heard the message of grace through faith, but his young mind couldn't comprehend beyond faith through right living, right thinking, right rule following. He stopped trying. It made it easier to walk away than seek truth.

Yet the religion of his youth also taught him the Bible. This Living Word was embedded in his subconscious, and he recalled it when he needed it most.

Two years after we were married, Scott had an accident resulting in extensive blood loss. Drifting in and out of consciousness in the ambulance, he experienced the weight of death without Jesus in his soul. He remembered these words from the Scripture reading of his youth: *Every knee will bow, every tongue confess, every knee will bow, every tongue confess, every . . . Jesus, save me! Jesus, save me!*

He was remembering the words of Philippians 2:9–11: "God also has highly exalted Him and given Him the name which is above every name, that at the name of Jesus every knee should bow, of those in heaven, and of those on earth, and of those under the earth, and that every tongue should confess that Jesus Christ is Lord, to the glory of God the Father."

That night, Scott was changed. He now had a *before* and an *after.* In between was the moment of his salvation, the moment of being saved by Jesus.

The transformation in my husband was something I couldn't

explain, and this transformation ultimately led to my own *before* and *after*.

Have you rejected Jesus Christ as Lord and Savior because of religion? Or perhaps have you mistaken religion for a personal relationship with Jesus Christ? Maybe you were like me in that season of life, considering Jesus to be a story like Santa Claus and the tooth fairy. Or has life brought you to this moment and you consider yourself beyond redemption, beyond God's mercy?

If this makes you wonder, *Am I prepared to die? Am I confident of my destination?* then please lean into what I am about to write. Friend, the Holy Spirit, who whispered to me in my *before*, lives within me now. He may be within you or beside you right now as you read.

God can bring beauty from ashes. In chapter 11, we learned the power of forgiveness and that faith, hope, and love were built on blood-drenched ground in Rwanda. If God can do that for a country, then he can also do it for you.

Know that you are here in this moment for a reason. The God of the universe and creator of all loves you so much that he will pursue you until your final breath.

> The Lord is not slack concerning His promise, as some count slackness, but is longsuffering toward us, not willing that any should perish but that all should come to repentance. (2 Peter 3:9)

Because this is true, I anticipate heaven will be populated by many who are there because of God's "longsuffering," or patience.

He pursued me too. I had to run to the end of myself before I realized that my soul would never be satisfied by the things of this world. I have shared my testimony many times in written word, from a stage, and one-on-one. However, not until that very moment, when Jesus saved me in my misery of miseries, did I realize that I didn't fully understand the gospel.

I understood the intensity of my own unworthiness, the sin embedded in my DNA, and the darkness of my soul without him. When I turned to him in complete desperation and repented, he responded by sending the Holy Spirit to reveal the meaning of the gospel and the centrality of the cross. And now I couldn't survive without him.

The Cross

If you or your loved one have received a serious or terminal diagnosis, you may be experiencing a multitude of emotions. Fear, trepidation, anxiety, and depression are common when we are faced with our own mortality. The unknown journey of dying may be the source of many of these. You may grieve your own death as you consider separation from those you love. But peace, joy, love, and *anticipation* can be found when you experience the hope found in the cross.

The cross is central to understanding the gospel. It is the place where God's righteous justice and infinite mercy reside. It is the place where death occurred and life was promised. It is the place of unimaginable despair and enduring hope. As a believer, the cross represents the death we deserve and reminds us of the cost that was paid for our healing. Without the cross, there would be no resurrection, and without the resurrection we could not *anticipate heaven.*

To understand the importance of the cross, we must understand why we need it. Let me give you an illustration I used on mission trips in Rwanda to explain the cross to children.

Our mission team often would set up stations outside the medical clinics we served. Under big tents, people enjoyed shade, water, and snacks, and these stations became places for laughter and games—which especially drew in children. And one of the games we played illustrates why we need Jesus.

We drew two lines in the dirt, approximately twenty feet apart. We lined up the children on one side and asked them to run and jump the expanse between the two lines. But it was way too far! No matter the physical ability of the child, none were able to jump such a distance.

We then sat down and described how we must view sin. On the other side of that distant line lives a perfect and holy God. He wants us to make it to the other side, to be close to him. But each of us who tries to make that jump will always fall short.

Earlier, before the children came, we had connected two long pieces of wood by rope to make a twenty-foot cross. It was great fun for everyone as children tried to jump farther than their friends and laughed when one of us would try and also fall short. They especially loved when our friend Andre Davis, an NFL record holder, tried and still couldn't make it across.

After everyone made their attempts to jump to the other side, we would gather together and bring out the cross and lay it across the great divide. The children could then walk across the cross as a bridge.

> Jesus said to him, "I am the way, the truth, and the life. No one comes to the Father except through Me." (John 14:6)

Jesus is the only way to enter the holy presence of the glory of God and the only bridge to the other side. He becomes more than the person we may have heard about as a child, more than a prophet believed in other religions, more than the person we read about, and more than just a "good dude" who had some "righteous" moments (okay, this came from a young surfer I once met).

Jesus died on that cross as the perfect Lamb of God. He bore our sin and experienced separation from his Father for the first time in eternity.

You might wonder, *How do we find hope in a story where Jesus dies?* The hope came three days later when death was conquered and Jesus Christ was raised from the grave to the right hand of the Father. *The hope is in the resurrection.*

> Blessed be the God and Father of our Lord Jesus Christ, who according to His abundant mercy has begotten us again to a living hope through the resurrection of Jesus Christ from the dead. (1 Peter 1:3)

Because of the resurrection, I anticipate that my death has been conquered, and he is the fulfillment of my living hope.

The Faith of a Child

Even the faith of a child, the faith to trust that walk on the cross to the other side, is a gift from God. If you find yourself just short of full faith in Jesus then, friend, pray for faith. The Son of God, who came to earth, died and was resurrected so we may have *forever with God in eternity.* God will deliver that last missing piece to show you the way. He does. Always. And as believers who have completed our faith walks, we must remember without death we would not experience the heaven we have anticipated. May we praise our way home!

> I say to you, ask, and it will be given to you; seek, and you will find; knock, and it will be opened to you. For everyone who asks receives, and he who seeks finds, and to him who knocks it will be opened. (Luke 11:9–10)

Accepting the truth of our own absolute spiritual poverty considering God's perfection creates in us a deep desire to seek him. When we receive the undeserved and miraculous gift of salvation, we are transformed. The Bible contains the words of God, and when we are transformed by the Holy Spirit, these words begin to leap from the pages into our hearts. They live and breathe within us, and we can understand them with greater clarity.

> For God so loved the world that He gave His only begotten Son, that whoever believes in Him should not perish but have everlasting life. For God did not send His Son into the world to condemn the world, but that the world through Him might be saved.
>
> He who believes in Him is not condemned; but he who does not believe is condemned already, because he has not believed in the name of the only begotten Son of God. (John 3:16–18)

When transformation occurs in the hearts of those who come to God in faith, death then becomes a lie. Jesus conquered death when he rose triumphant from the grave, and now this is his bold promise:

> Jesus said to her, "I am the resurrection and the life. He who believes in Me, though he may die, he shall live." (John 11:25)

Are *you* prepared to die? If you're not sure, then may today be the day you make your most important preparation. Since we began with Billy Graham and his bold question, let me share his written prayer of salvation to be your guide.

Dear God,
I know I'm a sinner, and I ask for your forgiveness. I believe Jesus Christ is your Son. I believe that He died for my sin and that you raised Him to life. I want to trust Him as my Savior and follow Him as Lord, from this day forward. Guide my life and help me to do your will. I pray this in the name of Jesus. Amen.[1]

And if you are sure, then take this moment to express your gratitude for the tender mercies you have been given.

> *Have mercy upon me, O God, according to Your lovingkindness; according to the multitude of Your tender mercies, blot out my transgressions.*
>
> PSALM 51:1

thirteen

A GOOD DEATH

Your place in Heaven will seem to be made for you and you alone, because you were made for it.

C. S. LEWIS

We began our journey together with the story of a patient who faced imminent death and yet comforted me with these words: "It's okay. I am going to have *a good death*." Even in her final days, she had anticipated heaven. She kept her eyes fixed on eternity throughout her earthly suffering, and it helped her declare her ending *good*.

We can do the same—but to finish each day, each season, each life *well*, we must create a spiritual practice. This is found in the final story and lasting legacy of my dear friend Lani.

In June 2017, I visited the famous Western Wall in Jerusalem. The cloudless sky was a brilliant blue. The place was packed with pilgrims who had come to pray. With my head covered out of respect for the traditions of this sacred place, I approached the women's side to pray with a friend who had been there before. In my hand I clutched a list of people I wanted to mention to God.

I stood there watching the people. Some rocked back and forth rhythmically. Others bowed their knees at this holy site where countless millions through the years have raised their voices and cried their tears. Not wanting to disrupt those who were wailing as they laid their hands on the wall, I took a few steps back and began to pray silently. When I finished, my friend gently reminded me of the custom. "You are supposed to touch the wall and leave your written prayer between the ancient stones." I remembered the small roll of paper with the names of those I prayed for that morning and pulled it from my pocket.

I stepped forward. As I did, I noticed that many of those praying were Jewish young women, some still in their teens. Some were weeping uncontrollably. Recognizing their deep emotions, I felt the urge to pray that God would respond to their heartfelt cries.

What happened next is hard to explain. As I reached out to touch the wall—the wall the Jewish people consider the holiest place on earth—I sensed the presence of God. It was as if it emanated from the wall and traveled up my arm to touch my heart.

My tears bubbled to the surface without conscious thought. The anguish of my soul flooded over me. Shame from a broken marriage, the pain of a son born blind, numerous losses, and assorted failures. I thought all these emotions had been solved, or at least buried deep enough that I no longer had access to them.

I am reminded of the apostle Paul's words to the Romans regarding the Spirit of God speaking on our behalf:

> The Spirit also helps in our weaknesses. For we do not know what we should pray for as we ought, but the Spirit Himself makes

> intercession for us with groanings which cannot be uttered. (Romans 8:26)

In those moments, I felt these heavy burdens rise to the surface of my consciousness. As the warmth of the wall traveled from my hands to my heart, I realized the Holy Spirit was reminding me that I had already been redeemed. But somehow it became a fresh reality, unexpected and cleansing.

How Long Do I Have?

On the prayer list I left in the wall in Jerusalem were the names of my dear friends Larkin and Lani Spivey. They were in their seventies, and they were still madly in love after forty-plus years of marriage. They had been healthy until Lani started to have some memory gaps. She brushed this off as part of aging, while Larkin and the kids were not so sure. Lani agreed to see a specialist.

These two were consummate planners and were well prepared for anything in life—except for the words, "Mrs. Spivey, you have a brain tumor. It appears to be a glioblastoma based on its pattern of growth."

Lani told me later that her first thought was, *Thank God! I finally have an explanation for the way I've been feeling.* Her first question was, "Can I pass this to my children?"

My friend Lani's life of caring for others came even in the moment of crisis. I can only begin to imagine the love that her devoted husband must have felt at that moment. I then imagine the fear he must have felt.

The question that came next is common when faced with stark images of mortality: "How long do I have?"

The doctor replied, "If it's what I think it is, probably less than two years."

That was on a Friday. When I returned home from Israel the following Monday, my husband, Scott, and I went directly to the Spiveys' home. Lani opened the door with her trademark smile and gave us a fierce hug.

She looked at me and laughed. "Ha! I'm going to get to heaven before you do!"

I broke out in tears and hugged her tighter. "Don't say that! We don't know what will happen." Over her shoulder, I could see a devastated family gathered around the table where they had previously shared so many celebrations. I thought of my prayers nestled in between the stones of the sacred wall in Jerusalem and wished I had been more specific.

On the way home, Scott and I were quiet, lost in our thoughts. I reflected on my friendship with Lani. How could I process life without her?

Lani had this great ability to look into a person's soul and speak the encouraging words most needed in the moment. She could somehow see the invisible qualities people possessed and the strengths that make them special, and she would name those things out loud.

Eleven years before my Western Wall moment, I had been in a dark, crushing season. Lani had seen my pain, drew near to me, and loved me unconditionally. She had walked with me every step of the way through that long chapter of my life.

All people everywhere need someone like Lani in their lives. She taught me to live in the moment but remember the heavenly future we are promised. She *anticipated heaven*.

Lani planned to share her Lord and Savior with as many people as possible after her diagnosis. She found this especially satisfying in loving and caring for the clinicians who were caring for her.

So in the summer of 2017, when Lani learned she had a brain tumor, people came in droves: friends with casseroles, friends to take her on slow walks, friends to sit with her, run errands, or do whatever she needed.

She went to the best doctors, and a biopsy confirmed the dreaded diagnosis. Radiation and chemotherapy were administered, with no response. It did not matter. Lani would sparkle when visiting with her doctors. She spread love to them even when she could no longer remember their names.

I took her for a ride one day in my convertible. She wore a scarf—expertly tied by her daughter—that covered her few remaining strands of hair. She enjoyed feeling the wind in her face, and we laughed about the movie *Thelma and Louise*, a favorite of ours.

Then Lani became serious. She told me she had been planning for the day when she would be gone. In fact, for at least a year, she had been going through closets and an attic filled with items she didn't want her children to have to deal with.

"I didn't even know then I was sick. I just felt I needed to do it. You do, too, Pamela. Don't leave all that stuff for your kids. They won't want it." She paused and added, "My dying has purpose. All the usual hurts and pains that families, especially big families, so often inflict on one another were resolved the moment my family heard about my tumor. When they came together, everyone was hugging and crying. I *loved it!* Wow, *that* was my miracle. I don't need to ask for another one."

Lani fought hard those first two months, I think mostly for her family. I was visiting one day and walked back to her bedroom, which was a beautiful place of quiet and peace. She was sitting in her bedroom chair with her eyes closed and cello music quietly playing in the background. Her scarf was in place, and her clothes were baggy on her tiny frame. On the dresser was a photo of Larkin and her when they were first married. What a striking couple they were.

I sat at her feet and placed my head on her hand, my tears falling to the floor. She patted my head, and I looked up at her. She didn't open her eyes but said quietly with a smile, "I love you. You know I am prepared, and Pamela, *I am so excited to meet Jesus!*"

Lani was comforted with the truth that in Jesus Christ, *death has lost its sting.* She knew we would see her again. She knew she would receive a heavenly body and would reside in a place without tears.

This beautiful planning woman ultimately had a dying plan. She was surrounded by her husband, children, and grandchildren in her earthly home while heading to her forever home. I can only imagine her reception there.

We Have a Choice

We can choose to see death as a curse, a dark power that binds us and those we love in fear. Or we can, in the face of death, do what Lani did: treasure the legacy—and memory—of a life lived well that results in a good death. Through it all, she anticipated heaven, and we can too.

My prayer for you and your loved ones as you have read *Anticipating Heaven* is that you are encouraged and feel equipped to navigate any diagnosis. The principles here will transcend health-care systems that evolve over time and place. This wisdom will give you choices for *what you want* for you, rather than *what others want.*

A *good death*, the declaration that inspired this book, is not an event; it is a *lifestyle*. As covered in these pages, it is a mind, body, and soul lifestyle that enhances life and changes the meaning of death.

As we conclude this time together, I hope you'll be empowered to care for your mind, body, and soul while you work through these difficult moments.

- For your mind, find peace in gaining knowledge, having a plan for the expected and unexpected, and diminishing the regrets you can change and laying down those you cannot.
- For your body, decrease suffering by asking the right questions at the right time, engaging the right services at the right time, and understanding that just because something *could* be done doesn't mean it *should* be done and may not be what you want.
- For your soul, pray for faith and encouragement, rest in the comfort of God's Word, and be refreshed in the quiet of your Lord's intimate presence. This daily practice will become the melody to help you praise your way home.

If we were together face-to-face, having a conversation about preparing for heaven, I'd end our time with a prayer. I'd take your hands and bow my head, wherever we were, and petition the Father for your peace and for the peace of those you love. That's how I want to leave you—with my prayer for you. And then, it's your turn. I invite you to lift your heart in prayer to the Father who guides, comforts, and leads home his children as they anticipate an eternity with him.

Dear Father God,

I come to you on behalf of those who have read these words. I pray for awareness of your intimate presence in their suffering and in their dying. I pray for your peace to replace chaos and fear. Dear God, touch them in the deepest part of their hearts where pain is a shadow that lingers. Lord, only you can heal their broken hearts, and only you can heal their broken bodies.

Dear Lord, please comfort the families who will temporarily lose sight of the one they love as you heal their physical bodies by giving them a spiritual body. Dear God, I cry out to you to wipe the tears and kiss the souls of those whose lives are marked by the grief of loss. Dear Lord, I pray that your goodness refreshes them even in the dark night of the soul.

Father God, I know that many pray at bedsides where the one who is falling to sleep has rejected your Son. Father, my prayer is that your endless mercy covers the families that grieve the eternal separation. Allow the Holy Spirit to move in those final hours, minutes, and seconds into the mind of the dying who have heard of you but still don't know you, who may have read these words and still denied you.

I pray that before their final breaths they called to you as Lord from the deepest recesses of their mind. If this, Lord, be your will, reveal to your saints that your Son knocked on the door of the one they love and in the stillness of their darkest night, he or she opened it and were welcomed home.

Dear Jesus, you paid our price; and now when God sees us, He sees you . . . and you are perfect. My Lord, may my life and these words glorify you and bring comfort to your children. Thank you for the opportunity to share in the lives of those who inspired this book and those who will one day read it.

Because of you, we will meet in heaven.

In your precious name,

amen.

> *Precious in the sight of the* Lord *is the death of his saints.*
>
> PSALM 116:15

ACKNOWLEDGMENTS

Thank you so much for taking a moment to read about the people who were so valuable in the development of this book. It is said "It takes a village to raise a child." It also takes a village to bring a book to fruition.

It has had many iterations and many talented and dedicated folks who believed in its mission and assisted me along the way.

I would like to begin with immense gratitude for Dr. John C. Maxwell, who wrote the Foreword and has written over a hundred books. His early encouragement after reading the manuscript kept me going. He has a personal commitment to share the gospel one-on-one to two hundred people each year, while also leading many to Christ as he speaks to thousands. He inspires me.

I would like to thank Jenny Harrington for bravely sharing through writing the story of her son Ewan's life and death from leukemia. His young life and death impacted many lives, including mine, in more ways than Jenny will ever know. Please consider donating to Seattle Children's Hospital in the name of Ewan Lill and the Team Ewan Guild to help fund cancer research for children. Visit www.seattlechildrens.org to give.

Dr. Jerry Pattengale and his wife, Cindy, were early readers and implemented the steps recommended. Dr. Pattengale is a prolific author (www.jerrypattengale.org) and winner of multiple awards and accolades, including four aces as a golfer. His books and articles have been an invaluable resource, as he is a master of his craft. He also seems to know everyone in Christendom and has been generous in sharing relationships that helped a budding author along the way.

The first was an introduction to Len Woods, a master writer and editor who gave advice on my first attempt at writing. Your impact on a writing generation will be felt. Thank you, Len.

He next introduced this book to Waverley Abbey College in the UK. Through many conversations and an epic trip to England, the title, *Anticipating Heaven,* was birthed by Dr. Micha Jazz. The CEO, Mark Markiewicz, and Dr. Jazz graciously allowed the mission of this book to take precedence over the ownership. They will be lifelong friends. During this England season, a very special editor, Joy McIlroy, was sidelined due to her own healthcare crisis. She remains in my prayers to this day.

Dr. Pattengale also introduced me to Johnnie Moore, President of JDA Worldwide, author, and world changer. Along with Ashton and Shelby, they helped bring to life my first published works. They were instrumental in teaching me the value of platform and introducing literary agent Bill Jensen to this work and to me.

I do not have adequate words to express my gratitude to Bill for the role he played in bringing this book to you. If it "takes a village," then Bill would be the mayor. His heart has been and will always be bringing the gospel to those who need to hear it. His mission is *the mission* of sharing the good news, and his words of wisdom and encouragement always came at the precise time I needed to hear them. Thank you to his wife, Sheila, who is the twinkle in his eyes and the skip in his step.

Thank you, Diane Woerner. Your heart for this mission, this

book, and the art of writing were instrumental in guiding and shaping the manuscript. Your skills as a writer and editor were invaluable to me.

Because of Bill I can thank my amazing publisher, W Publishing Group and Thomas Nelson. Thank you, Don Jacobsen, Damon Reiss, Carrie Marrs, and Caren Wolfe for choosing this book and its mission to become one of your missions.

Carrie has been the greatest encourager and a gift from God. In his mercy, he brought our lives together. Carrie, your story from your youth of caring for your mother is an example of why this book was written.

Carrie and her editing coworker Jenn McNeil taught me so much in the early editorial process, and their excellence in writing and editing, as well as their care for me, delighted my soul. Jen Stair guided it home, and Rachel Buller gave me a personal word of encouragement exactly when I needed it. The marketing team was exceptional in creative thinking and in capturing the heart for the mission of this book. Thank you, thank you!

A special thanks to the Five Wishes Foundation, their founder Jim Towey, and leadership Paul O'Malley and Ed Towey. Their commitment to caring for those who are facing the end of life is an inspiration for those who labor in this field and the patients they serve. My deepest gratitude for allowing me to share the Five Wishes Advance Care Plan, "the plan with a heart and soul."

On a personal note, thank you Dr. Charles and Florence Mugisha for founding Africa New Life Ministries and your spiritual mentorship. You taught me how to have a *reckless dream*. Alan, Natalie, Dan, Betty, and the rest of my Africa New Life Ministries family, thank you for your excellence on mission. It is an honor to work alongside you.

Joel, Laura, and Sayde Walker from www.launchmybook.com, thank you for your love, support, and wisdom.

Becky Fisher, my Kilimanjaro climbing sister and my Creative Executive Assistant, has literally been the wind beneath my wings. Tatum, her niece with Munives Marketing, brought a youthful perspective to the conversations her generation is having around faith, dying, and death. I could not have asked for a better creative team. Shout out to Betty for bringing us together.

My friends David and Lisa Horsager prayed for this book, and David, a *New York Times* bestselling author, taught me so much about the value of trust through his many books.

I also want to thank my friends who picked me up when I needed it and always brought laughter to our gatherings. Kelli, Nancy, Melanie, Debbie, Julia, Susan, Teri, Jodie, Renata, and Amanda, *muchas gracias*!

Jodie Wert, you were a godsend when I needed it at the beginning.

Christine Soules, you are the lift in my heart when I need it most.

Rebecca Hagelin, your life intersecting with mine reminds me of God's intimate love and tender mercies.

Dad and Denise, thank you for your loving support. Mom, you are the best and thank you for *always* being my cheerleader.

Finally, I want to thank my family—my husband, Scott, and each of my children—who paid a price for the long hours I worked and the commitment that comes from being a doctor. The wisdom gained from patients through the years required extra time, and it came at a cost to my family. In many ways, *this book is rightly yours*. Amber, Brooke, Britney, Zander, and Christian, I'm sorry I wasn't a better cook, but, so proud of how you each thrived despite it and have gone on to chase your own dreams.

FURTHER PRACTICAL RESOURCES

This collection of resources has been curated to help you take your next steps in preparing for heaven and your departure from this earth. In it you will find:

Resource A: When Decisions Should Be Shared
Determining when you or a loved one needs assistance with decision-making

Resource B: Guide to Documents and Advance Planning
Names and uses of common legal and personal planning documents

Resource C: Understanding Brain Death
Solid facts to guide you through a fearful time

Resource D: Understanding Persistent Vegetative State
Facts on an often misunderstood diagnosis

Resource E: Planning for Peace Checklist
Practical tasks to complete while anticipating heaven

Resource F: End-of-Life Timeline Signs and Symptoms
Exactly what to expect at the end

Resource G: The Dictionary of Serious Illness Terms
Terms you may encounter at the hospital

Resource A

When Decisions Should Be Shared

No matter where you are in your health journey, if you have intact decision-making capabilities, it is never too late nor too early to begin this process of planning for a day when you are not able to make decisions for yourself. Your decision-making now determines your autonomy in the future. You are choosing times when your healthcare proxy or designated loved one will begin to assist you with choices for your health. It is far preferable to participate in your own plan rather than rely upon others to intervene due to safety.

What should you do if your loved one is already experiencing difficulty with decision-making? This may be a time when you utilize closed-ended questions with the patient. For example:

"Dad, we need to have a plan of care that Bob and I can use to help you when the doctor feels you may need some assistance. I know you want to stay in your house, but to do so we must have a plan. Do you want to discuss this now, or set a time on Saturday?"

This is a nonthreatening approach. You are not taking anything, you are acknowledging that he or she has choices, and you are defining what is important to decide. Decide together what benchmarks or goals are needed to determine if he or she can stay at home. You are preparing for the discussion around a detailed plan. With permission from the patient, you can enlist the doctor's advice and support for a plan.

Achieving a goal of choosing a healthcare proxy is very important in this circumstance. It will allow you to talk with the doctor about your concerns and perhaps initiate an evaluation for dementia.

A primary care provider will most often refer a patient to a neurologist for mental-status exams and determination of competency.

Even for people in the prime of life, these decisions can be complicated. How much more so when we begin to age and experience common mental lapses? Understand there is no shame in this; it happens to the best of us and to some degree all of us.

Four criteria or abilities have proven to be useful benchmarks for determining when a person may need help in making important healthcare decisions:[1]

Understanding. This is the ability to comprehend the information that is being disclosed regarding one's current condition. Can the patient offer a description of their mental/physical state in their own words that is consistent with their actual condition?

Appreciation. This is the ability to apply relevant information to oneself and the current situation. For example, in the case of patients with mild dementia, can they appreciate the facts that (a) their disease process is starting to inhibit their ability to make decisions for themselves and (b) that the discussion at hand is for the purpose of determining how much this is already taking place?

Reasoning. This is the ability to think rationally and logically, to understand the consequences of one's actions. Can the patient solve simple problems or apply information to practical life situations?

Expression of a choice. This is the ability to verbalize clear decisions and to communicate one's desires effectively. Can the patient make their wishes known in an understandable way?

When do we find ourselves using these criteria? Usually on behalf of someone else. And most commonly when we notice negative consequences. For example, an elderly patient continues to drive despite getting lost frequently or having frequent fender benders. Or, when a patient is either unable or unwilling to make medical choices (often because they do not fully understand the consequences). For example, a patient might refuse to take needed medications.

Remember this distinction: *decisional capacity* is a clinical term; *decisional competency* is a legal term, determined by a court.

For patients: this is my best counsel and strongest encouragement for you, the patient, if you are noticing memory loss or other difficulties that may impair your capacity to make good decisions.

- Talk to your doctor. First, engage your clinician in these hard "crossroads conversations." A clinician should be able to assist you in determining when it is time to assess when you may need to be evaluated. He or she may refer you to a neurologist, psychologist, or psychiatrist with more experience in assessing these matters.
- Understand your wishes. How would you like to spend your last chapters if you have been diagnosed with early or mild dementia?
- Explain it to your family. Help your family understand what is important to you and how to maintain your independence while still engaging your family in the process.

For caregivers and loved ones: it would be wonderful if your loved one, the patient, was proactive and followed the steps above to initiate the conversation. In reality, you as the loved one may be making it for them. Here are my recommendations.

- Talk to the doctor. Make an appointment to speak with your loved one's doctor. He or she might not be able to discuss the clinical status of the patient, but they may listen to your concerns. If you cannot schedule an appointment, write a letter with your concerns and hand-deliver it.

- Accept the patient's wishes. If the patient has been determined to have intact decisional capacity and is simply making choices that are not in line with what family members desire, you must be prepared to accept their decisions. I find this most often in situations where elderly parents have lived independently for decades, are still thinking clearly, yet are becoming frail. Adult children want Mom and/or Dad to change their living situation, and parents don't want to leave their home. This is where "aging in place" conversations are helpful and where all parties need to agree the quality of their loved one's final days means much more than the number of them.
- Explain it to the family. It is crucial that all family members understand and agree with the process that is taking place. Otherwise, undue stress will be placed on the patient from having to process everyone's different opinions on his or her status. Sadly, I have witnessed too many arguments between family members (sometimes standing around the patient's bed!) as they argued over "what Mom wants." Often, this is what *they* want for Mom, not what Mom wants. In every instance, this kind of conflict is not what Mom needs.

A day will come when decisions need to be made and shared. Be prepared in advance. One approach that I used in my family is whatever choices my mother and I agreed on, I also agreed to for myself. Therefore, my children will know if the time comes, when to share in my decision-making.

Resource B

Guide to Documents and Advance Planning

Advance Directives

We have used the term advance care plan or ACP throughout this book. Advance Directives (ADs) are the component documents of the plan. The Five Wishes is most represented in the Combined Directive. These documents define preferences for medical care in the event the patient is unable to make decisions or speak on their own behalf. These written wishes serve to direct family members and healthcare providers during difficult, stressful, and sometimes end-of-life situations.

Advance Directives address the following:

- **Living Will:** This legal document addresses questions about one's desire for life support or other life-extending medical procedures in the event one is incapacitated and/or at the end of life. It is legally binding. Multiple topics are covered in a living will. Usual components of the living will include instructions regarding:
  - **CPR:** CPR (cardiopulmonary resuscitation) is an attempt to save life in the event one's heart or one's breathing stops. This can include chest compressions, electrical shocks to the heart, medications, fluids, and mechanical ventilation.
  - **Mechanical ventilation:** The use of a machine to take over the work of breathing for a patient because of low oxygen levels or in the event of needed airway protection because of an allergic attack or being comatose.

- **Tube feeding:** The provision of nutrition through a tube that is placed through the nose or, when prolonged periods are expected, directly into the stomach through the abdominal wall.
- **Dialysis:** The use of a machine to replace kidney function, a process that removes waste from the blood and helps manage a proper balance of electrolytes and fluids in the body.
- **Antibiotics or antiviral medications:** Medicines utilized to treat infections.
- **Comfort care:** The provision and management of a patient's comfort when further treatment of a disease has ceased.
- **Organ and tissue donation:** Living wills offer the opportunity to specify one's desire to donate his or her vital organs. (Note: Donors who are on life support cannot be removed from life support until organ procurement has occurred.)
- **Donation of one's body:** The desire to "leave my body to science" can also be expressed in a living will.

- **Durable Power of Attorney for Healthcare:** This legal document, also known as a *healthcare proxy* or *healthcare power of attorney*, designates a surrogate decision maker if a patient is unable to make decisions on their own behalf. This individual can be a family member, trusted friend, clergy member, or attorney. He or she needs to have a clear understanding of his or her role and must be willing to carry out the requests set forth in the patient's living will. Common identifiers for this individual are *healthcare agent*, *healthcare proxy*, *healthcare surrogate*, *healthcare representative*, *patient* *advocate*, or *healthcare attorney-in-fact*. If such a person has not been designated, then each state in the United States has a legal policy for the definition and appointment of a surrogate, generally beginning with a spouse, followed by adult children, siblings, and so on. There are also state-by-state policies for patients without family or designated friends and for circumstances in which guardianship is appointed on behalf of the patient. A clinician or caseworker generally refers the patient to the court system in circumstances such as this.

- **Combined Directive:** A combined directive includes the above two documents plus a *values history*. A *values history* gives more explicit directions for what a person wants at the end of life based on emotional desires, spiritual beliefs, and physical circumstances. An example of a combined directive would be the Five Wishes document. Clinical conditions covered under a combined directive could include everything from a coma with virtually no chance of recovery, a coma with a small chance of recovery, to a probable impaired state, advanced dementia, or advanced dementia with a terminal illness.
- **Physician Orders for Life-Sustaining Treatment (POLST):** These are medical orders signed by a clinician that delineate what care is to be delivered based upon the desires expressed by the patient during an advance care planning (ACP) discussion. You may ask your clinician or the provider who is assisting you with your ACP if POLST documents are legal in your state and if you should have them. While Do Not Intubate (DNI) and Do Not Resuscitate (DNR) orders are included within the framework of POLST orders, these are not all the decisions that can be ordered within POLST. The

purpose of POLST is to have a consistent continuum of care across all healthcare settings so the patient's wishes are met in each possible scenario.

For an effective POLST program, there must be consistency in a coordinated effort of care, which is called the *POLST paradigm.* To see if your state has legal policy regarding POLST, review the United States map at www.polst.org.

Hopefully these definitions and descriptions bring clarity to the terms used in ACP. If you are currently under a doctor's care for any reason, it is a reasonable expectation to have your healthcare provider or his or her designate review the components of an ACP and make recommendations to assist you in making a living will. For Medicare and Medicaid recipients, as well as those covered under certain private insurance plans, the costs associated with consulting your doctor(s) about these matters are reimbursed.

Resource C

Understanding Brain Death

There *is* consensus in the medical community about the criteria for brain death, but there is *not* always consistency in how these criteria are assessed and applied in different real-life situations.

Here is my advice to anyone who has a loved one on life support and who hears discussions regarding brain death.

- Understand that it is a complex process to diagnose brain death. On October 11, 2023, consensus guidelines were published.[2] While these guidelines are described in medical terms, the process can still be understood. For example, the doctor will complete various tests to confirm the absence of brain function. One of these tests is called an *apnea test*, in which they stop artificial respiration and determine that the patient does not breathe on his or her own.

- Confirm the appropriate clinicians have determined brain death before drawing any definitive conclusions or making any decisions.
- Insist that all necessary examinations (neurologic and apnea tests, and so on) be performed and all recommended observation periods be followed.
- Know that the clinician determining brain death should not be the attending physician and should not be a member of an organ transplant team.
- Understand that once a patient is declared brain dead, that patient is no longer legally living. Brain death is death. This has been determined by Part 2 of the Uniform Determination of Death Act.[3] This "extends the common law basis for determining death—total failure of the cardiorespiratory system . . . to include the new procedures for determination of death based upon irreversible loss of all brain functions."

This is an extremely difficult circumstance for families. A body that is kept alive by machines may still look alive. But unlike a patient that is in a coma and on machines, the brain has no electrical activity and therefore no function. This is incompatible with any definition of life. As a family member or healthcare proxy, you will not be asked to stop machines. Clinicians are required by law to stop them if the patient meets criteria for brain death. However, most clinicians will allow time for family to be with the patient before they do. If a patient is a candidate for organ donation, the discussion will take place before machines are stopped.

Resource D

Understanding Persistent Vegetative State

Persistent vegetative state is a complex diagnosis. The diagnosis is based upon clinical features and the phrase "not likely to recover." This phrase is dependent on the time from onset of the persistent vegetative state, and what caused it.

If the patient experienced a prolonged period without oxygen to the brain, "not likely to recover" can be diagnosed after three months of observation. If the cause is due to brain trauma (for example, from an accident), the time required for a clinical diagnosis of "not likely to recover" extends to twelve months. For family members, it is usually difficult to comprehend this diagnosis. The following features are invariably present in someone "not likely to recover":

- intact sleep-wake cycles (natural rhythms of sleep and wakefulness)
- loss of self-awareness
- lack of purposeful response to external stimulation (no meaningful response to external stimulation)
- inability to communicate
- lack of comprehension when spoken to
- inability to focus on objects with eyes and sometimes eyes moving independently of each other
- occasional nonpurposeful limb movements, noises, facial grimaces, or smiling

- area of the brain called the brain stem that controls the heart, breathing, and temperature regulation functions to a variable degree (unlike brain death, where none of these functions are present)[4]

The most important things to remember in this situation are (a) the time required before a clinical diagnosis can be made, and (b) that life support in this circumstance is most often the use of a feeding tube. Patients still have brain stem function and therefore should eventually be able to breathe on their own. In many circumstances, this only leaves decision-making around the use of a feeding tube. ACPs address feeding tubes and will help families and healthcare proxies determine what the patient would want.

Resource E

Planning for Peace Checklist

The following checklist breaks down end-of-life planning into categories, providing handy to-dos based on discussions in this book. It also includes additional planning that leads to peace for the patient. (Family members and loved ones, as you review this list, please consider engaging in the areas in which the patient may need help.) It is not meant to overwhelm you, but it is a comprehensive resource you can keep returning to as you implement one item after another. Regardless of your age or health status, beginning this plan early prepares you for the expected and unexpected.

Don't worry if some of the terms seem unfamiliar. The list is followed by a Discussion Guide, explaining new terms *in italics* and expanding on each category. I recommend scanning the list, reading the Discussion Guide, and then returning to check off each category one by one.

HEALTHCARE

- ❑ Medical Records Digital Access Instructions
- ❑ Medical Care Contacts List
- ❑ Medical Records Summary File
- ❑ Advance Care Plan (see chapters 5–7)
- ❑ POLST Form (see page 202–203)
- ❑ *Aging Location**
- ❑ Palliative Care Preferences
- ❑ Hospice Care Plan
- ❑ *End-of-Life Doula**

RELATIONSHIPS

- ❑ Restoration Plan*
- ❑ Call Tree (see page 149)
- ❑ Care Plan (for spouse or other relationships if you have been the primary caregiver, parent, or guardian)
- ❑ Domestic Partner Agreement*
- ❑ Caregiver Team
- ❑ Pet Care

PRACTICAL MATTERS

- ❑ *Ethical Will**
- ❑ Last Will and Testament
- ❑ *Legacy Plan**
- ❑ *Giving Plan**
- ❑ *Estate Plan**
- ❑ *Swedish Death Cleaning**
- ❑ *Donation Strategy**
- ❑ Asset List
- ❑ Bank Accounts
- ❑ Debts

DOCUMENTS

- ❑ Insurance Policies
- ❑ Titles and Registrations
- ❑ Social Security Card
- ❑ Employment History and Dates
- ❑ Military History
- ❑ Contracts
- ❑ Loan Documents, including those Paid in Full
- ❑ Medicare/Medicaid/Other Health Insurance Cards
- ❑ Policies or Prepaid Plans Covering Funeral Expenses
- ❑ Driver's License
- ❑ Passport
- ❑ Birth, Death, Wedding Certificates
- ❑ Name Change Documents
- ❑ Divorce Settlement Documents
- ❑ *Family History**
- ❑ All Other Documents Included in the Other Categories of this Checklist

CONTACTS

- ❑ Personal
- ❑ Professional—Attorney(s), Financial Adviser, Accountant
- ❑ Executor of Will

ACCOUNTS AND PASSWORDS

- ❑ Email
- ❑ Computer
- ❑ Cell Phone/Tablet/Other Devices
- ❑ Subscriptions
- ❑ Credit Cards
- ❑ Airline and Hotel Reward Accounts
- ❑ Store Accounts
- ❑ Medical Accounts

- ❑ Financial Accounts
- ❑ Insurance Accounts
- ❑ Music/Video/Internet/Television/Cable/Phone Accounts
- ❑ Professional Accounts
- ❑ Donation Accounts
- ❑ Automatic Food Delivery/Amazon/Grocery Delivery (instructions for cancellation of automatic deliveries)
- ❑ Social Media Accounts
- ❑ Recurring Payment Accounts

DIGITAL DEATH

- ❑ Digital Assets List (defined in the discussion guide)
- ❑ Authorization (giving authorization access to your chosen individual for your digital asset list discussed in the guide)
- ❑ *Digital Mourning**

END-OF-LIFE PLAN

- ❑ Funeral Plans
- ❑ *My Last Six Months**
- ❑ *Living Wake**

Discussion Guide for Planning for Peace Checklist

Healthcare

Medical Records Digital Access

Most large medical facilities and some doctor's offices have online access to patient records. These are called patient portals. You can ask at the facility where you receive care if they have this feature. You will want to give your healthcare proxy and other people of your choice instructions on how to access the portal. There are often verification measures included when the patient portal is set up. This may be a text, an email confirmation, or security questions.

- Doctor's Office
- Hospital
- Imaging Center

Medical Care Contacts List

- Physicians—Primary Care, Specialists, Consultants, Hospice, Dentists
- Insurance—Photocopies of ID Card, Name, Phone Number, Address
- Ancillary Services—Physical Therapy, Occupational Therapy, Home Health Providers, Pharmacy, Hospice Nurse, End-of-Life Doula*

Medical Records Summary File

You should keep a hard copy of your healthcare summary. You may request a summary from your primary care physician, the hospital at times of discharge, skilled nursing facilities, assisted living facilities, and hospice facilities. Also, keep copies of your Advance Directives, Do Not Resuscitate Forms, and POLST forms if available (see Resource B).

Aging Location

Specify your preference: age at home, or age elsewhere?

- Age at Home: Aging at home or in a home setting with caregiving provided by family, home healthcare, medical assistants, in-home care sitters, hospice care.
- Aging Elsewhere: Aging in assisted living, skilled nursing, or other group settings.

Palliative and Hospice Care

- **Palliative Care:** A multidisciplinary approach to medical care for those living with serious illnesses. You can choose ahead of time which local provider you'd like to receive palliative care from.
- **Hospice Care:** A multidisciplinary approach to achieve comfort and quality of life for those approaching end-of-life, which is defined as when a disease course is expected to end within six months. You can research ahead of time to determine your preferred hospice care company or facility in your area.
- **End-of-Life Doula (Death Doula):** These nonmedical care providers give additional support, education, and comfort for those facing death or even fears associated with death. They work closely with family and hospice providers to advance support for the individual and those who care for them. Currently, their services are not covered by insurance. Fees vary by provider, and some doulas donate their time for their service. I would recommend the International End-of-Life Doula Association as a starting point to determine if hiring a doula is what you need for your circumstance. They also have a search tool to identify end-of-life doulas in your area. Their website is www.inelda.org.

Relationships

Restoration Plan: A plan to rebuild relationships through forgiveness and reconciliation with those who are important to you and whom you would want to include in your dying process. Healing through forgiveness and reconciliation brings peace and comfort when you need it most. Identify those relationships in your life that keep you up at night or that you wish you still had when you need them most.

Call Tree: You will need help from those closest to you to complete a call tree. If you or your family need to activate the call tree, only one call will need to be made rather than many to relay information, prayer requests, and visiting schedules. I describe this in more detail in "How to Build a Call Tree" in chapter 10.

Care Plan: A plan of care for those in your life who depend on you for their care or special needs. Activating this plan early will ease your burden at a time when you need care. It is best to seek legal counsel if the patient is mentally incapacitated or an underage child.

Domestic Partner Agreement: This is a legal document prepared for individuals who live together as partners but are not married by law. Its terms are highly variable based on the circumstance.

Caregiver Team

Whether you live alone or have a large family, it is important that you know who your caregivers will be and that they know their roles as caregivers. This will include your healthcare proxy, professional providers such as hospice, and your home support team, which may include family, friends, neighbors, and others.

Pet Care

- Short-term—for hospital stays, trips out of town, or staying in homes filled with people who may be allergic.
- Long-term—if you are unable to care for your pet on a permanent basis, or in the event of your death. Our pets feel like family, and it will be important for you to know your family will be cared for well, including your pet.

Practical Matters

Ethical Will

An *ethical will* is a personal, nonlegal document designed to transfer values, memories, and what are considered meaningful teachings from one generation to another. Its origin is found in Jewish tradition and the Hebrew word *zava'ah*. It is considered a living document that can be started at any point in life.

Last Will and Testament

A *last will and testament* is a legal document that transfers tangible assets in the event of your death. Depending on your assets, this can be completed independently, through online sources, or with an attorney.

Legacy Plan

A legacy plan is a personal document that may be included within an ethical will but should also be considered an independent document. We each leave a legacy, sometimes good and sometimes bad. However, those who create a legacy plan desire to be intentional with the legacy they leave. Understand that legacy may be composed of one or many values and valuables. For example: A family value of caring for the poor with the financial valuable of 10 percent of income. Or a spiritual valuable of teaching Scripture beginning in youth, and the family value of a biblical worldview.

Giving Plan

A *giving plan* often parallels a legacy plan. A giving plan can be initiated at any time in life. It begins with a statement of why to give and the value of giving. For our family, our giving plan is based upon the biblical scripture Malachi 3:10: "'Bring the whole tithe into the storehouse, that there may be food in my house. Test me in this,' says the LORD Almighty, 'and see if I will not throw open the floodgates of heaven and pour out so much blessing that there will not be room enough to store it.'"

We often consider financial resources as our only wealth to be considered for intergenerational wealth transfer. However, I want you to consider that anything you give for the benefit of others carries wealth. Your life and the wisdom gained from experience is a valuable gift for generations to come.

The structure of a giving plan may be as specific as to delineate giving percentages to chosen ministries or causes. However, more importantly, it aligns with the legacy plan and creates processes for vetting where resources go to align with your family values.

Estate Plan

An estate plan is a collaborative document between you, your family, financial adviser, accountant, tax attorney, and other professionals serving in the area of estate planning. Everyone does not need an estate plan; however, understanding if you need one is essential.

Estate planning can begin early in life. Estate planning

generally requires expertise in a multitude of disciplines. Some firms specialize by consulting in these areas. I would recommend a trusted relationship with your financial adviser who, with the right team, can maximize your income, your impact, and your wealth for future generations. When you align your last will and testament or trust, your estate plan, your giving plan, and your legacy plan, you will experience deep peace from the order that comes with a plan.

Swedish Art of Death Cleaning

Döstädning, or "death cleaning," is a Swedish methodology of decluttering. This results in benefits for your immediate family. And most who complete a Swedish death cleaning process find it beneficial for themselves. As they declutter in action, they feel unburdened in emotion. And who does not want be a little less burdened? A book titled *The Swedish Art of Gentle Death Cleaning* by Margareta Magnusson is a good read on this topic.[5]

Donation Strategy

Where will your stuff go after you're gone? For the things you don't leave to loved ones, donate. Evaluate your local charities for donating clothing and other nonvaluable items. My advice is to choose one and determine if they can arrange pickup for your convenience. I have personally worked with Goodwill, the Salvation Army, and Habitat for Humanity. But there may be smaller charities in your area that would benefit. I would consider women's shelters, homeless shelters, and foster care nonprofits.

Asset List

To help your inheritors, make a list of valuables, including:

- Money
- Bank Accounts—Savings, Checking, CD, Money Market. Take note that these accounts can avoid probate by changing to *Payable on Death* or *Transfer on Death* accounts with a named beneficiary. Ask your bank about this.
- Cash on Hand—if large sums are kept and stored
- Gold/Silver
- Real Estate
- Home (include mortgage holder if applicable)
- Secondary Properties
- Investment Properties
- Business Properties
- Investments (include accounts such as stocks and bonds)
- Retirement Plans (these should not be included in a will, as you specify the beneficiary with the fund)
- Digital Assets (include cryptocurrency, non-fungible tokens, websites, branding, copyrighted items, trademark ownership, emails and email accounts, metadata, documents, music libraries, and other assets with potential monetary value)

Beneficiary Accounts

These may include insurance policies, pensions, or retirement accounts. These should be included in your asset list, but not your will. This will avoid their delay through probate court.

Businesses

Any business either wholly or in part owned should have a succession plan in writing, including handling of assets. This should be discussed with an attorney.

Personal Valuables

Include anything of financial value or sentimental value for which you desire a specific designation upon your death. This includes jewelry, art, collections, cars, and so on.

Debts

List all loans, including personal loans that must be attended to in the event of your death. Include loan location, account, approximate amount owed, and payoff date. If possible, discuss with your loan officer the process that occurs in the event of your death. Consider all financial costs associated with end-of-life care, funeral and burial, probate court costs, and care for loved ones, and plan for that from your available assets.

Documents

Keep originals in a fireproof box with instructions for access in another location. Alternatively, you can keep your documents in a safe-deposit box that at least one other person is added to for easy access. Keep copies in a secondary folder that is easily accessible.

End-of-Life Plan

This incorporates all else not covered and is primarily meant for your last six months of life. It describes what is important for you to do during this time and how you will find comfort.

Your end-of-life plan may include plans for a living wake, a time to celebrate you and your life. Loved ones say good things about you, like they would in a eulogy, except you are there to hear them. It is a valuable time to say your goodbyes.

It also will include a funeral plan. The experts in the funeral industry will guide you through the process. Taking part in the planning process gives you the opportunity to speak to your loved ones after you are gone.

Consider an online digital program for end-of-life planning with options to upload the documents. Also, many times a financial adviser will have platforms such as eMoney for digital storage of important items. The most important aspect of any online data storage is protection of your documents. Security measures should be easily identifiable and understandable.

Contacts

Professional: It is always good to keep a handwritten or printed document that is an easily accessible list of your professional contacts. While this may seem old-fashioned, it circumvents any technology failure in the event you or your family need important numbers quickly. These may include physicians, home health agencies, hospice agencies, attorneys, financial advisers, workplace relationships, business partners, and so on. You should also include a digital contact in your contacts list and always include the individual's role in the company name line of the contact card so that this will be easily accessible. More detailed information can be included in the notes section.

Personal: Ideally, you sync all your contact lists into one digital location and make sure you write down where this list is located. The article "How to Organize Your Messy Contacts List" does a very nice job of explaining the variety of options and which is the best option.[6] You may also have a traditional handwritten address book or a digital file of your Christmas card list; keep this with your other important documents.

Accounts and Passwords

Digital password keepers with encrypted security are invaluable in the safekeeping of this important information. Rather than keeping up with multiple passwords, you only need to maintain separately the master password.

There are many individuals who are not comfortable keeping anything stored online (my mother included). If this is your choice, then make sure a list of passwords to your digital accounts is stored with your documents in a fireproof box or safe-deposit box, and let your trusted individual(s) know how to access it. At least one other person should be on the safe-deposit account to access in the event you are unable.

Digital Death

We live our lives with increasing interface in a digital world. Online, many of our lives have expanded far beyond our immediate family, friends, workplace, and communities. We can be proactive in managing our online presence in the event of our death, including email, phone access, social media accounts, and more. Because things change so rapidly in the digital world, my advice is to search online for the topic *digital death* for an up-to-date plan.

Digital Mourning

It is a relatively new use of social media to post end-of-life messages, memorials, and grief sharing.

Resource F

End-of-Life Timeline Signs and Symptoms

Here is what you can expect as the body lets go and death is imminent.

One to Three Months Prior to End-of-Life

- Diminished appetite
- Increased sleeping
- Increased pain and nausea
- Increased risk of infections
- Weight loss
- Possible apathy or introspection
- Less active
- Less communicative or a desire for deeper meaning with communication

One to Two Weeks Prior to End-of-Life

- Greater desire to sleep
- Increased lethargy
- Possibly stop eating
- Sometimes increased restlessness
- Increased oral secretions
- Increased chest congestion
- Increased confusion
- Increased hallucinations or visions, often involving loved ones who have passed (death awareness)
- Fluctuating temperature, blood pressure, and respirations
- Fluid buildup in gravity dependent areas

Days or Hours Before End-of-Life, Often Called *Active Dying Phase*

- May experience a sudden or brief surge of energy and clarity of thinking and speech
- Declining blood pressure
- Loss of bowel or bladder control possible

- Erratic breathing
- Possible agitation
- Extremities cold, mottled, and sometimes purple or blue
- Eyes may remain half-opened and teary
- Breathing sounds wet (death rattle)
- Near Death Awareness (see page xx)
- Patients still hear despite being unconscious

Minutes to Moments Before End-of-Life

- Expect eyes and mouth to be partially or fully opened
- Expect gasping breathing
- Weak or fluttering pulse

Resource G

The Dictionary of Serious Illness Terms

- **Cancer:** A disease that occurs when normal cellular death does not occur and abnormal cell division and growth results in further dysregulation and, ultimately, disease.

  If you are diagnosed with cancer, your most important resource of unbiased information can be found on the website www.cancer.gov. For a complete listing of cancer terms, see the following web page: www.cancer.gov/publications/dictionaries. Additionally, on the website www.clinicaltrials.gov you can research ongoing trials for which you may be a candidate.
- **Cancer staging:** This is a process used to determine the extent of one's cancer. It is based on different factors depending on the type of cancer and if it has spread. The stage determines the types of treatment available. While the cancer

may change during treatment or after, it is always identified by its original stage and a modifier reflecting any change. For detailed information on staging, review the following website page: www.cancer.gov/about-cancer/diagnosis-staging/staging.

- **Metastasis:** This is when tumor cells spread from the original site.
- **Prognosis:** Many factors determine prognosis. When you request prognosis information, generally the physician will give you a prognosis based on statistics gathered from a large number of people who have your cancer type in the stage that you have. It is vital to understand other factors specific to you and the genetics of your cancer also determine your prognosis. The following are terms that you may hear regarding the statistical prognosis:
    - **Cancer-specific survival:** This is also called *disease-specific survival* and refers to the percentage of patients with a specific type and stage of cancer who have *not* died from their cancer during a certain time period after diagnosis. Benchmark times are generally one year, two years, and five years.
    - **Overall survival:** This is the percentage of people with a specific type and stage of cancer who have *not* died from any cause during the same benchmark times.
    - **Disease-free survival:** This is also called *recurrence-free survival* or *progression-free survival* and reflects the percentage of patients who have no signs of cancer during a certain period of time after treatment.
    - **Cure:** This is an absolute statement that there are no traces of your cancer, and the cancer will never come back.

- **Remission:** The signs and symptoms of your cancer are reduced. This can be labeled as partial or full remission.

Machines and Other Medical Equipment and Procedures

Some of these terms are explained in Resource B, however, I will review key components that you may hear.

Lungs and Respiration

- **Mechanical Ventilation, Ventilator, Artificial Respiration, Breathing Machine:** These are the names of therapies and devices that do the work of breathing for a patient by placing a tube through the mouth into the lungs for delivery of oxygen and pressure. These machines and procedures provide various levels of assistance for patients depending on their needs. When the patient improves, they are "weaned" from the machine. Depending on the circumstance, most patients will have a daily weaning trial. This is sometimes called "a sedation vacation," meaning the sedative that the patient is on is decreased to determine whether the patient is capable of having spontaneous respirations on his or her own. This determines whether the patient can be weaned. If the patient has very low oxygen levels, he or she is not a candidate for weaning. Healthcare providers will still do a sedation vacation to assess mental status while off medication.
- **CPAP or BiPAP:** This is a breathing assist device that uses a mask to deliver oxygen and pressure to expand the lungs.
- **Arterial Blood Gas (ABG):** A test that measures oxygen,

carbon dioxide level, and acid/base status in a patient. It requires drawing blood from the patient, typically from an artery in the wrist.

- **Pulse Oximeter:** A clip placed on the patient's finger that shows the percentage of oxygen in the blood.
- **Endotracheal Tube (ETT):** The tube you may see in a patient's mouth that is connected to the ventilator. It delivers oxygen to the lungs as opposed to the stomach.

Cardiovascular (Related to the Heart Vessels)

- **Basic Life Support (BLS):** This is training in basic measures of CPR. I highly recommend that everyone take this short course and certification program that is offered by the Red Cross, local fire departments, and hospital systems around the world. This is the first line of defense if a person has difficulty breathing, is choking, or becomes unconscious.
- **Advanced Cardiac Life Support (ACLS):** This is training required of emergency medical technicians (EMTs), for example, the "ambulance heroes," and all other clinicians who care for patients in ERs or hospital settings.
- **Automatic External Defibrillator (AED):** These are compact machines that determine a patient's heart rhythm and automatically determine if a low voltage electrical current or "shock" should be delivered in an attempt to return the heart rhythm to normal. They are typically found in high-traffic areas such as airports and malls.
- **IV:** This is the acronym for *intravenous* and is plastic tubing that delivers fluids and/or medications through a patient's vein.
- **Central Line:** This is an IV line inserted into a large vein in the neck or under the clavicle or "collarbone" so that specific

medicines and fluids can be given. Central lines must be watched carefully for risk of infection.

- **PICC line:** This is the acronym for *peripherally inserted central catheter* and is a type of central line inserted into the arm. These can be used for longer periods of time (up to months) for administering medications such as antibiotics or chemotherapy.
- **Shock:** Unlike the "shock" associated with a defibrillator, this is when a patient's blood pressure is abnormally low for reasons such as sepsis (severe infection beyond the original source), cardiac (the heart not pumping strongly enough), blood loss, hypovolemic (severe dehydration), hypothermic (dangerously low body temperature), and so on. Treatment is aimed at identifying the cause, giving fluids (unless cardiac), and medications to either improve heart function (if cardiac) or to increase blood pressure.

Nutrition and Gastrointestinal (Food and Stomach)

- **Nutritional Supplement:** Taken orally or through a feeding tube. A feeding tube can be short-term (through the nose into the stomach) or long-term (via a PEG Tube, G Tube, or J Tube—each variety identifying the tube's location, such as in the stomach or first part of the small intestine). The most important thing is that these can be used long-term for delivering nutrition. The short-term options are for when a patient is on a ventilator or post-op recovery and the goal is to start nutrition as quickly as possible. This is a part of healing. The long-term use of intestinal feeding has many more indications; however, also more complexities. This is one of the areas where even the best advance care plan (ACP) may not be the right plan for the circumstance. Understanding your options or options for those you proxy is crucial.

- **Total Parenteral Nutrition (TPN):** A nutritional option given through either a central line or a PICC line (a type of central line in the arm). For example, for a patient with severe pancreatitis, when the primary treatment is not eating, TPN is sometimes used while the pancreas heals. TPN is a short-term solution for nutrition because of risk of infection if used long-term.

The Patient Journey: Words You Need to Know

- **Hospital Observation vs. Admission:** Hospitals and clinicians are closely regulated when a patient is admitted to the hospital. In the majority of cases, patients are admitted under observation status (which can be up to forty-eight hours). To be admitted (not observation status), specific criteria must be met by a diagnosis, needed treatment, or unstable vital signs or labs. For the patient, the treatment will be the same. However, as a patient (or a family member of one requiring hospitalization), make sure that you understand if you are being admitted or are under observation and how this will affect your discharge planning. You can ask to speak to a case manager if within twenty-four hours one has not visited you. Why is this important? Certain post-hospitalization benefits are only available if you meet the requirements for admission under Medicare/Medicaid guidelines, such as home health or home physical therapy. I must emphasize that it is not at a physician's or hospital's discretion to determine admission vs. observation (although previously it was). The point is to begin planning for hospital discharge from the moment you enter so that you are adequately prepared.

- **Home Healthcare vs. Home Care:** Although I have listed the main web page in the Resources, the most comprehensive explanation for the differences between home healthcare and home care can be found at: www.mymedicarematters.org/2018/03/help-need-home-assistance-options/. Home healthcare consists of medical professionals that typically follow you after a hospital stay until you are stable. Home care may consist of nonmedical care providers or medical assistants who stay for extended periods of time with patients. If you are not on Medicare or Medicaid, it is important to know the details of medical insurance coverage. All the fine print that no one likes to read is *critically important* when it comes to the paradigm shifts, especially when it comes to home healthcare and home care. Knowing what benefits that you have and do not have will help guide you in your decision-making process. Paradigm shifts do not always come with the warning, "Here I am to take you out of work for a while/a long time/forever."
- **Short-Term Disability vs. Long-Term Disability** insurance policies are available. As you would imagine, these policies are less expensive when you are young and healthy, but they cannot be purchased when illnesses, acute or chronic, have already been diagnosed.
- **Social Security Disability:** One of the most complicated, illogical, log-jammed government services I have ever encountered. I routinely treat fully functional patients who are receiving full disability benefits. I know they are able to work

because they *do* work for cash on the side. (Note: You are *not* supposed to qualify for disability assistance if you can work.) I treat other patients who desperately need disability benefits yet are denied multiple times in a process that can sometimes take years before getting approved. Some attorneys specialize in helping people through this incomprehensible maze. If you can find a good one (be careful, because there are some con artists out there) to help you navigate all the red tape and rejection that you are likely to encounter, you are fortunate, indeed. Know that even if you succeed, disability payments are generally much lower than one's working income.

- **Long-Term Care Insurance:** There are many nuances to these policies, but a good insurance agent can walk you through them. This is worth looking into.

Final Wishes

During the final paradigm shift, the important words involve what you do not want done more than what you do want done:

- **DNI:** All ACLS measures are utilized except an endotracheal tube for a mechanical ventilator.
- **DNR:** This specifies that when a patient experiences cardiovascular collapse or respiratory failure, he or she does not want ACLS measures. He or she only wants to be made comfortable in those final moments. If a patient is on a ventilator already and a healthcare proxy and physician recognize the patient meets requirements that would fall into the DNR parameters, this means ACLS will not be initiated if the patient worsens, although all other current measures will be continued.

- **Comfort Measures Only:** In the case of an actively dying patient, the patient (via an advance directive) or his or her proxy may request hospice to expertly manage the issues around comfort. For example, if a patient were on a ventilator, the tube used for breathing on the machine would be removed and only comfort medicines would be administered. This would include morphine for pain and shortness of breath, benzodiazepine (such as Ativan) for anxiety, scopolamine for excess secretions, acetaminophen for fever, and other medications depending on the circumstances. Comfort at home also includes the guidance of a hospice nurse and medical equipment such as hospital beds, bedside commodes, and wheelchairs.

Palliative Care

- Patient does not have to have a time-limiting terminal diagnosis.
- Patient is living with chronic disease.
- This focuses on relief from suffering.
- Patient can continue to use life-prolonging medications.
- A multidisciplinary approach to care is started, including meeting the patient's physical, mental, social, and spiritual well-being. It is appropriate in all stages of disease that are chronic.
- Treatment is most often through physician offices, hospitals, and occasionally at home if homebound.
- This should be considered in nearly all paradigm shifts if a patient has a chronic disease that affects *activities of daily living (ADLs)*. Check with your insurance carrier, or discuss with your clinicians.

Hospice Care

- Must have a terminal diagnosis.
- Patient is not expected to live longer than six months. This determination is made by a clinician who follows specific parameters to refer a patient to hospice. Comfort Measures Only is implemented for the *disease-defining illness.* This means no lifesaving therapies administered (for example, no chemotherapy or radiation other than radiation for pain management). But if the patient is hospitalized for a reason other than the terminal disease, Medicare will cover with your regular coverage. An example of this was the patient who had prostate cancer but was admitted post–cardiac arrest.
- **Care coordinators** are generally hospice nurses with oversight by a hospice physician. Care can be administered at home, occasionally at a "hospice home," or in the hospital if the patient is expected to die within two weeks of removing life-support machines.
- **Combined Care:** The majority of palliative care providers are also hospice providers. The best of circumstances is to begin palliative care and then transition to hospice care when it is appropriate.

NOTES

Chapter 2: An Unanticipated Reality

1. Robert J. Sullivan, Lawrence W. Menapace, and Royce M. White, "Truth-Telling and Patient Diagnoses," *Journal of Medical Ethics* 27, no. 3 (2001): 193, https://www.ncbi.nlm.nih.gov/pmc/articles/PMC1733397/pdf/v027p00192.pdf.
2. Adapted from "Questions to Ask About Your Cancer," American Cancer Society, accessed March 2, 2024, https://www.cancer.org/content/dam/cancer-org/cancer-control/en/worksheets/questions-to-ask-about-my-cancer.pdf.
3. J. R. R. Tolkien, *Return of the King* (New York: Houghton Mifflin Harcourt, 1954), 951–52.

Chapter 3: When in a Foreign Land

1. If you, or someone you love, has been diagnosed with mild cognitive impairment dementia, or another illness that may make decision-making difficult, refer to Resource A: When Decisions Should Be Shared.
2. H. O. Mauksch, "The Organizational Context of Dying," in Elisabeth Kübler-Ross, *Death: The Final Stage of Growth* (New York: Simon and Schuster, 1975), 17.
3. Mauksch, "The Organizational Context of Dying," 17.
4. Anne Carrie, "The 8 Most Common Root Causes of Medical Errors," *Always Culture*, June 28, 2022, https://alwaysculture.com/hcahps/communication-medications/8-most-common-causes-of-medical-errors/.

5. "Find and Compare Providers Near You," Medicare.gov, https://www.medicare.gov/care-compare/.
6. Shu-Fen Niu et al., "A Comparison of the Effects of Fixed- and Rotating-Shift Schedules on Nursing Staff Attention Levels: A Randomized Trial," *Biological Research for Nursing* 15, no. 4 (October 2013): 443–50, https://doi.org/10.1177/1099800412445907.
7. Anton N. Isaacs et al., "Hospital Medication Errors: A Cross-Sectional Study," *International Journal for Quality in Health Care* 33, no. 1 (2021): 1–6, https://doi.org/10.1093/intqhc/mzaa136.
8. Adapted from "Choosing Wisely," American Board of Internal Medicine, https://abimfoundation.org/what-we-do/choosing-wisely.
9. "Patients' Bill of Rights," US Office of Personnel Management, https://www.opm.gov/healthcare-insurance/healthcare/reference-materials/bill-of-rights.
10. You can also report a specific complaint related to patient safety if the hospital is accredited by the Joint Commission, considered the highest level of accreditation. Its website is www.jointcommission.org.

Chapter 4: Diminishing Chaos

1. Victor Fleming, dir., *Gone with the Wind* (Selznick International Pictures, 1939), DVD.
2. Marilyn J. Field and Christine K. Cassel, eds., "Approaching Death: Improving Care at the End of Life," *Institute of Medicine (US) Committee on Care at the End of Life* (Washington, DC: National Academies Press, 1997), https://pubmed.ncbi.nlm.nih.gov/25121204/.
3. Marla J. Silveira, Scott Y. H. Kim, and Kenneth M. Langa, "Advance Directives and Outcomes of Surrogate Decision Making Before Death," *New England Journal of Medicine* 362, no. 13 (April 2010): 1211–18, https://www.nejm.org/doi/full/10.1056/nejmsa0907901.
4. Silveira, Kim, and Langa, "Advance Directives and Outcomes."

Chapter 5: A Bargain and a Treasure

1. Five Wishes, https://www.fivewishes.org.

Chapter 6: The Hard Hard Choices

1. Emily Galassi Sullivan et al., "Familiar Auditory Sensory Training in Chronic Traumatic Brain Injury: A Case Study," *Disability and Rehabilitation* 40, no. 8 (2018): 945–51, https://www.tandfonline.com/doi/full/10.1080/09638288.2016.1277403.
2. Stephen Ashwal et al., "Medical Aspects of the Persistent Vegetative State," *New England Journal of Medicine* 330, no. 21 (May 1994): 1499–1508, https://www.nejm.org/doi/full/10.1056/nejm199405263302107.

Chapter 8: Paradigm Shifts: Anticipating Heaven in the Storm

1. Louis Lasagna, "The Hippocratic Oath: Modern Version," *Nova*, PBS, https://www.pbs.org/wgbh/nova/doctors/oath_modern.html.
2. "About Chronic Diseases," Centers for Disease Control and Prevention, accessed May 15, 2024, https://www.cdc.gov/chronic-disease/about/index.html.
3. "International Classification of Functioning, Disability and Health (ICF)," World Health Organization, 2001, https://www.who.int/standards/classifications/international-classification-of-functioning-disability-and-health.
4. Andrew J. Cutler, "Managing Physical Illness and Depression," *Psychiatric Times*, August 29, 2013, https://www.psychiatrictimes.com/view/managing-physical-illness-and-depression.
5. Amy Fiske, Julie Loebach Wetherell, and Margaret Gatz, "Depression in Older Adults," *Annual Review of Clinical Psychology* 5 (April 2009): 363–89, https://doi.org/10.1146/annurev.clinpsy.032408.153621.
6. *Social Isolation and Loneliness in Older Adults*, National Academies of Sciences, Engineering, and Medicine (Washington, DC: The National Academies Press, 2020), https://doi.org/10.17226/25663.
7. Reinhold Niebuhr, *Book of Prayers and Services for the Armed Forces* (New York: Federal Council of Churches, 1951).

Chapter 9: The Final Paradigm Shift: "Wow, This Is It!"

1. "Hospice Facts and Figures 2024," www.thenationalallianceforcareathome.org, September 9, 2024, https://www.nhpco.org/wp-content/uploads/NHPCO-Facts-Figures-2024.pdf.

2. Ava Kofman, "Endgame: How the Visionary Hospice Movement Became a For-Profit Hustle," ProPublica, November 28, 2022, https://www.propublica.org/article/hospice-healthcare-aseracare-medicare.
3. Palliative and hospice care in countries other than the United States will most likely have different regulations but will have a governing board. The internet provides easy access for evaluation of hospice and palliative care centers, and most will have a national association similar to the United States.
4. Adam Marks and Lucille Marchand, "Near Death Awareness," Palliative Care Network of Wisconsin, February 11, 2019, https://www.mypcnow.org/fast-fact/near-death-awareness/.
5. April Mazzarino-Willett, "Deathbed Phenomena: Its Role in Peaceful Death and Terminal Restlessness," *American Journal of Hospice and Palliative Medicine* 27, no. 2 (2009): 127–33, https://doi.org/10.1177/1049909109347328.
6. Marks and Marchand, "Near Death Awareness."
7. Mazzarino-Willett, "Deathbed Phenomena."
8. Madelaine Lawrence and Elizabeth Repede, "The Incidence of Deathbed Communications and Their Impact on the Dying Process," *American Journal of Hospice and Palliative Medicine* 30, no. 7 (2012): 632–39, https://doi.org/10.1177/1049909112467529.

Chapter 10: The Power of Prayer in God's Sovereign Care

1. "Sepsis Fact Sheet," Sepsis Alliance, revised August 2023, https://www.sepsis.org/sepsis-basics/what-is-sepsis/.
2. Harvard University, "Prayers Don't Help Heart Surgery Patients; Some Fare Worse When Prayed For," ScienceDaily, April 3, 2006, www.sciencedaily.com/releases/2006/04/060403133554.htm.
3. Jeff Levin, *God, Faith, and Health: Exploring the Spirituality–Healing Connection* (New York: John Wiley and Sons, 2001), 181–204.
4. Richard P. Sloan and Rajasekhar Ramakrishnan, "Science, Medicine, and Intercessory Prayer," *Perspectives in Biology and Medicine* 49, no. 4 (2006): 504–14, https://doi.org/10.1353/pbm.2006.0064.
5. LaPrincess C. Brewer et al., "Religiosity/Spirituality and

Cardiovascular Health: The American Heart Association Life's Simple 7 in African Americans of the Jackson Heart Study," *Journal of the American Heart Association* 11, no. 17 (August 2022), https://doi.org/10.1161/JAHA.121.024974.

6. James W. Anderson and Paige A. Nunnelley, "Private Prayer Associations with Depression, Anxiety and Other Health Conditions: An Analytical Review of Clinical Studies," *Postgraduate Medicine* 128, no. 7 (2016): 635–41, https://doi.org/10.1080/00325481.2016.1209962.
7. Allen C. Sherman et al., "A Meta-Analytic Review of Religious or Spiritual Involvement and Social Health Among Cancer Patients," *Cancer: An International Interdisciplinary Journal of the American Cancer Society* 121, no. 21 (November 2015): 3779–88, https://doi.org/10.1002/cncr.29352.
8. Jeff Levin, "Prevalence and Religious Predictors of Healing Prayer Use in the USA: Findings from the Baylor Religion Survey," *Journal of Religion and Health* 55, no. 4 (August 2016): 1136–58, https://doi.org/10.1007/s10943-016-0240-9.
9. "New Testament Greek Lexicon (NAS)," Bible Study Tools, "sozo," https://www.biblestudytools.com/lexicons/greek/nas/sozo.html.

Chapter 11: Hope amid Suffering

1. "Rwanda Summary," *Britannica*, accessed September 27, 2024, https://www.britannica.com/summary/rwanda.
2. Bridge2Rwanda website, http://www.bridge2rwanda.org/.
3. "Mother Teresa Quotes," *Catholic Online*, accessed May 14, 2024, https://www.catholic.org/clife/teresa/quotes.php.

Chapter 12: The Most Important Preparation

1. "Start Your New Life with Christ," Billy Graham Evangelistic Association, https://lp.billygraham.org/find-peace-with-god/.

Further Practical Resources

1. Thomas Grisso and Paul S. Appelbaum, *Assessing Competence to Consent to Treatment: A Guide for Physicians and Other Health Professionals* (New York: Oxford University Press, 1998); L. H. Roth,

A. Meisel, and C. W. Lidz, "Tests of Competency to Consent to Treatment," *American Journal of Psychiatry* 134, no. 3 (March 1977): 279–84, https://doi.org/10.1176/ajp.134.3.279.

2. New York State Department of Health, "Guidelines for Determining Brain Death," revised November 2023, https://www.health.ny.gov/professionals/hospital_administrator/letters/2011/brain_death_guidelines.htm.
3. Michael Nair-Collins, "The Uniform Determination of Death Act Is Not Changing. Will Physicians Continue to Misdiagnose Brain Death?" *The American Journal of Bioethics*, July 2024, 1–12, doi:10.1080/15265161.2024.2371129.
4. Stephen Ashwal et al., "Medical Aspects of the Persistent Vegetative State," *New England Journal of Medicine* 330, no. 21 (May 1994): 1499–1508, https://www.nejm.org/doi/full/10.1056/nejm199405263302107.
5. Margareta Magnusson, *The Gentle Art of Swedish Death Cleaning* (New York: Scribner, 2018).
6. Whitson Gordon, "How to Organize Your Messy Contacts List," *New York Times*, June 18, 2019, https://www.nytimes.com/2019/06/18/smarter-living/organize-google-apple-phone-contacts.html.

ABOUT THE AUTHOR

DR. PAMELA PYLE is a board-certified internal medicine physician and has practiced medicine for over three decades in United States hospitals and in nascent communities throughout Rwanda. She serves as chair of the board for Africa New Life Ministries, serves on the White Flag Medical Advisory Board, and is a Museum of the Bible Woman of Legacy.

She speaks and writes nationally and internationally on the topics of evangelism, women's discipleship, health equity, healthcare, and end-of-life care.

Her website, www.drpamela.com, is a resource for navigating the foreign world of healthcare by uniting medicine and faith to bring wisdom and hope.

Pamela is a wife, mother to five, grandmother to eight, adventurer, author, poet, and "Reckless Dreamer." She and her husband, Scott, call South Carolina and an airplane seat their home on the way to fulfilling their purpose. For more resources, visit www.drpamela.com.